# THE DEPENDENT PERSONALITY

# THE
# DEPENDENT
# PERSONALITY

ROBERT F. BORNSTEIN

THE GUILFORD PRESS

NEW YORK / LONDON

© 1993 The Guilford Press
A Division of Guilford Publications, Inc.
72 Spring Street, New York, NY 10012

Printed in the United States of America

This book is printed on acid-free paper.

Last digit is print number: 9 8 7 6 5 4 3 2 1

**Library of Congress Cataloging-in-Publication Data**
Bornstein, Robert F.
    The dependent personality / Robert F. Bornstein.
      p.   cm.
    Includes bibliographical references and index.
    ISBN 0–89862–991–8
    1. Dependency (Psychology)   2. Personality disorders.   I. Title.
    [DNLM: 1. Dependency (Psychology)   2. Dependent Personality
Disorder.   BF 575.D34 B736d]
    RC569.5.D47B67   1993
    616.85'8—dc20
    DNLM/DLC
    for Library of Congress                                    92–49466
                                                                    CIP

Permission to reprint in this volume substantial portions of "The Dependent
Personality: Developmental, Social, and Clinical Perspectives" by R. F.
Bornstein, 1992, *Psychological Bulletin, 112,* 3–23 is gratefully acknowledged.
© 1992 by the American Psychological Association. Reprinted by
permission.

*To Mary*

# *Acknowledgments*

A number of people contributed in important ways to the completion of this book. I could not have written *The Dependent Personality* without their help and support. First and foremost, I would like to thank my research assistants: Linda L. Baker, Karen R. Cornell, Amy R. Kale, Michelle L. Koons, Amy B. Krukonis, Carla C. Mastrosimone, Kathleen A. Manning, and Stephanie C. Rossner. Their help in conducting literature searches for this book made an overwhelming project a bit less overwhelming. Among them, my students spent dozens—if not hundreds—of hours poring over indexes of psychological and medical research, conducting computer searches of the psychological and medical literatures on dependency, and tracking down journal articles and book chapters. They made the entire project come together.

I would also like to thank Susan R. Roach and Nellie R. Heller, Senior Library Specialists at Gettysburg College. Their ability to locate and obtain obscure books and journal articles that were needed for this review was critical in allowing me to complete the book. During the course of this project, I needed to obtain many books and journal articles that were not available in the Gettysburg College library. These requests were often made using incomplete—and, on occasion, incorrect—information. Nonetheless, virtually every interlibrary loan request that I made during the course of this project was fulfilled.

I am very grateful to Seymour Weingarten, Editor-in-Chief of Guilford Publications, for his enthusiastic and unwavering support of this project from its earliest stages. Without his encouragement, I would not have written this book.

Finally, I would like to thank a number of colleagues who commented on earlier drafts of *The Dependent Personality*. Kathleen M. Cain, Paul R. D'Agostino, Jeffrey G. Johnson, Joseph M. Masling, Richard M. O'Neill, Jack D. Shand, Stephen M. Siviy, and Joel L. Weinberger gave generously of their time and energy, reviewing chapters of this book and offering many valuable suggestions for revision. *The Dependent Personality* was greatly improved as a result of their input.

# Preface

During the past 40 years there has been an enormous amount of research examining the etiology and dynamics of dependent personality traits in children, adolescents, and adults. In a sense, researchers' interest in this topic is not surprising: Dependency is a ubiquitous psychological phenomenon—a universal life experience. In infancy, every one of us was completely dependent on our primary caretaker for protection, nurturance, and support. Moreover, those of who are fortunate enough to live to a ripe old age may find that we leave life much as we entered it—dependent on others for help, protection, and guidance.

Between adolescence and old age, most of us are as autonomous and independent as we will ever be. However, some of us are more independent than others. Even in adulthood, certain people continue to show exaggerated dependency needs. Such people have traditionally been described as having a "dependent personality." As the ensuing chapters will show, a dependent personality orientation affects an individual's behavior in a wide range of situations and settings. Thus, dependency has been of interest to psychologists whose work touches on a variety of topics and issues.

It is possible to get a sense of the degree to which researchers have been interested in studying dependency by obtaining a rough estimate of the number of journal articles published on this topic during the past several decades. A thorough search of the psychological and medical literatures revealed that more than 500 empirical studies of the dependent personality have been published since 1950. This total does not include the hundreds of theoretical articles and case studies that also appeared during this period. Furthermore, researchers' interest in dependency continues to increase with each passing year. Between 1950 and 1959, there were about 60 published studies investigating aspects of the dependent personality. From 1960 to 1969, that figure doubled, and there were more than 120 published studies in this area. Between 1970 and 1979, there were more than 130 published studies of the dependent personality, whereas the period from 1980 to 1989 saw more than 160 articles on this topic. Interest in dependency shows no signs of waning: During 1990 and 1991 alone, there were more than 40 published studies in this area.

I believe that a volume reviewing and integrating the empirical literature on dependency is now needed, for two reasons. First, there has never been a thorough, detailed review of the empirical literature on dependency and the dependent personality. Second, although developmental, social, and clinical psychologists share an interest in dependency, there has been relatively little integration of the findings that have emerged in different areas. More often than not, researchers investigating a particular aspect of dependency show little awareness of findings from other research domains. This book was conceived with the aim of filling these two gaps. The purpose of this book is to review the empirical literature on the antecedents, correlates, and consequences of dependency. My goal is to link developmental, social, and clinical research programs in this area in order to arrive at a broader, more integrated perspective on dependency and the dependent personality.

Although the actual writing of this book took place during 1991 and 1992, the impetus for *The Dependent Personality* dates back to 1981, to my first day of graduate work in the Clinical Psychology doctoral program at SUNY–Buffalo. I had been assigned to be Dr. Joseph Masling's research assistant as part of my graduate fellowship. When I found Joe's office and introduced myself, I discovered that he already had several studies planned for us, one of which was an experiment investigating the relationship of oral dependency to sensitivity to nonverbal cues. We ran the study during the Fall 1981 semester. It bombed. Nonetheless, my interest in dependency was kindled, and during the next several years Joe Masling and I conducted a number of studies examining the dynamics of dependent personality traits. I continued to work in this area during my predoctoral internship year at the Upstate Medical Center in Syracuse, New York, and during my first few years of teaching at Gettysburg College. However, I was increasingly bothered by how disconnected the field of dependency research had become. It seemed to me that the time had come for someone to pull together what we had learned about dependency during the past 40 years, and to write an integrative review of the empirical literature in this area.

During the summer of 1990, I began to work on such a review. My intention was to write a *Psychological Bulletin*–type article reviewing the empirical literature on dependency and the dependent personality. By the end of 1990, I had in hand a finished draft of the paper. The article was eventually published, and I believe that it provides a very useful overview of this area of research (see Bornstein, 1992). Unfortunately, journal page limitations prevented me from discussing a number of interesting and important topics in this review article. Thus, after my initial review was published, it seemed clear to me that there was more to be done in this area. So, using my initial ideas as a foundation, I expanded my review of the empirical literature on dependency. That expanded review became this book. My views regarding the etiology and dynamics of dependency have changed considerably since my original review article was published. In retrospect, I have come to view my *Psychological Bulletin* paper as an initial effort to make sense of a complex and wide-ranging area of research. This book represents the culmination of my efforts in this area—the final product of a decade of theoretical and empirical inquiry.

*The Dependent Personality* is divided into ten chapters. It is worth taking a moment to describe the content and structure of these ten chapters in order to place the ensuing material into the proper context.

The first two chapters of *The Dependent Personality* provide information regarding the various conceptual and theoretical frameworks that have influenced research on dependency, and they discuss some of the methodological difficulties involved in measuring and studying dependent personality traits. Thus, in Chapter 1 I describe the most influential theoretical models of dependency, and discuss in detail the various definitions of dependency that have been utilized by developmental, social, and clinical psychologists. In Chapter 2 I provide an overview and critique of commonly used measures of dependency, contrasting the strengths and weaknesses of objective, projective, behavioral, and interview-based dependency scales.

In Chapter 3 I review studies that examine the etiology and development of dependency in infancy, childhood, and adulthood. This chapter not only provides an opportunity to survey the empirical literature on the acquisition and development of dependent personality traits, but also allows for a comparison of the predictive validities of two important theoretical frameworks: the psychoanalytic and social learning models of dependency.

Chapters 4 and 5 present contrasting and complementary views of the influence of dependency on social behavior. Dependency is, by definition, a trait that is manifested primarily in interpersonal interactions. However, the effects of dependency on interpersonal behavior take two distinct forms, and studies of these two aspects of dependency are discussed separately. In Chapter 4 I review research on the interpersonal consequences of dependency (i.e., the effects of dependency on social behavior), and in Chapter 5 I review research on dependency as a social cue (i.e., the effects of dependency on others' responses and reactions).

In Chapter 6 I review research on dependency and psychopathology. This is the longest chapter in the book, and its length reflects the tremendous amount of time and energy that researchers have invested in studying the dependency–psychopathology relationship during the past several decades. Chapter 6, like Chapter 3, affords me an opportunity to compare directly the predictive validities of the psychoanalytic and social learning models of dependency.

Chapters 7, 8, and 9 deal with more narrowly defined, focused areas of research than are dealt with in some of the earlier chapters. In Chapter 7 I discuss research on Dependent Personality Disorder, a diagnostic category that is now just over a decade old. In Chapter 8 I review research on the relationship of dependency to risk for physical disorders, a topic that has long interested psychological and medical researchers. In Chapter 9 I review studies of dependency and patient-related behaviors (e.g., compliance with treatment regimens). Chapter 9 also provides an opportunity to connect empirical findings regarding the influence of dependency on behavior in social settings with some empirical findings that examine the effects of dependency on behavior in clinical settings.

Finally, in Chapter 10 I discuss and integrate findings from developmental, social, and clinical research in order to get as complete a picture as possible of the traits and behaviors that compose the "dependent personality" in children and adults. In this chapter I present a new theoretical model of dependency that emerges from the findings reviewed in Chapters 3–9, and discuss the implications (and practical applications) of this model.

In writing *The Dependent Personality*, I discovered that different topics and issues seemed to warrant somewhat different treatments. For example, the approach that worked well for describing developmental research on dependency was inappropriate for discussing research on Dependent Personality Disorder. Similarly, the framework that I used to evaluate social research on dependency just didn't work when I reviewed studies of dependency and physical disorders. Thus, I chose to use somewhat different approaches in different chapters, rather than being bound to one particular approach throughout the book. Some chapters focus primarily on empirical studies on a particular topic (e.g., Chapters 4 and 6), while other chapters involve more extensive theoretical discussions (e.g., Chapters 3 and 8). In some chapters I review the empirical literature in the traditional narrative format (e.g., Chapters 2 and 9), while in other chapters meta-analytic and quasi-meta-analytic techniques are used to uncover hidden patterns in the empirical literature (e.g., Chapters 5 and 7).

Despite these differences, there are some common threads that run through all the chapters in this volume. In every chapter, I tried to include an extensive review of the empirical literature, including the most recent findings on a particular topic. I critique relevant empirical studies in each area, pointing out conceptual and methodological limitations in particular investigations. In every chapter, some discussion of historical trends is included in order to place recent (and not-so-recent) findings into the proper context. In addition, I attempted to summarize the state of the art in each area of research that I reviewed, pointing out which issues have been addressed conclusively, and which questions require additional study. As much as possible, I tried to integrate the material discussed in different chapters by noting parallels among the research findings that have emerged in different domains, as well as by pointing out those areas wherein different investigations have produced inconsistent, conflicting, or puzzling results.

After considerable thought, I decided to include in this review a number of studies that had relatively serious methodological flaws and limitations. One could argue that it would have been better to limit the review to those studies that were methodologically and conceptually airtight. However, it seemed to me that there are several advantages to providing a comprehensive review of the dependency literature—a review that presents this literature exactly as it is, warts and all. First, some studies provided important information regarding the dependent personality despite having significant flaws and limitations. Second, a discussion of the conceptual and methodological weaknesses of research in this area is important in a historical sense, insofar as these weaknesses have a great deal to say about the ways that investigators approached thorny empirical questions at various points in the history of dependency research. Third, comparison of the findings obtained in flawed studies versus studies that were methodologically and conceptually more rigorous can, in and of itself, provide important information regarding the etiology, dynamics, and correlates of dependency. Thus, in the end I decided that the benefits of providing a comprehensive review of the dependency literature outweighed the costs of including in the review some less-than-perfect studies.

*The Dependent Personality* focuses primarily on studies that examine individual differences in dependency. Studies that assess the effects of variables that exacerbate or ameliorate dependent feelings (e.g., social isolation) but do not include an individual difference measure of dependency are not discussed. In addition, I did not include in this review extensive discussions of the literature on several topics that are, to varying degrees, related to dependency. For example, although there is some overlap between the concepts of dependency and "insecure attachment," it was clear that a thorough review of the attachment literature was beyond the scope of this book. Thus, I discuss the dependency–attachment relationship only briefly, focusing on those studies that are most relevant to questions regarding the etiology and dynamics of dependent personality traits.

Similarly, although there is some overlap between the concept of dependency and constructs such as field dependence, institutional dependence, learned helplessness, need for affiliation, and need for approval (i.e., social desirability), I chose to include in this book only those investigations in which individual differences in dependency were assessed directly. Related topics and overlapping constructs are discussed only when they have important implications for our understanding of the antecedents, correlates, and consequences of dependent personality traits.

This volume is intended for two audiences. First, the book should be of interest to researchers interested in personality development and dynamics, in social cognition and behavior, and in the etiology and psycho-dynamics of psychopathology. Thus, developmental researchers—especially those interested in social and personality development—should find *The Dependent Personality* to be of interest. Similarly, social psychologists whose work touches on such dependency-related topics as affiliation, conformity, compliance, and prosocial behavior may find this book valuable. Finally, clinical researchers should find this volume to be useful, particularly those sections of the book that deal explicitly with psychopathology and treatment issues.

Second, this book will be of interest to practitioners, because clinical work invariably involves dealing with issues related to dependency. In fact, the concept of dependency is central to much of clinical psychology, counseling, social work, and psychiatry. Dependency is inextricably linked to transference and countertransference dynamics, to the dynamics of the supervisory relationship, to the psychological processes associated with psychiatric hospitalization and discharge, and to psychotherapy initiation and termination. To the extent that the clinician is informed regarding the most recent empirical findings regarding the dependent personality, his or her ability to deal productively with dependency issues as they arise during diagnostic, testing, therapeutic, and supervisory activities will be enhanced.

# Contents

# Dependency in Context: Conceptual and Theoretical Frameworks

Although psychologists have long been interested in the antecedents, correlates, and consequences of dependent personality traits, no single widely accepted definition of dependency has yet been described. Neki (1976a) traced the linguistic roots of the term *dependency*, concluding that it was originally derived from the Latin *dependere*, which, roughly translated, means "to be suspended or hang down." As Neki (1976a) noted, "pejoration can be seen embedded in the very root meaning of dependence" (p. 2). Ainsworth (1969) similarly noted that dependency in adults invariably "implies immaturity" (p. 970). Siegel (1988) was more direct in her assertion that "dependency is devalued and pathologized. It is linked with symbiosis, weakness, passivity, immaturity and is attributed to women, children, and persons perceived as inadequately functioning" (p. 113). Although Birtchnell (1991a, 1991b) and others (e.g., Alexander, 1970; Bowlby, 1969; Henderson, 1974; Woolams & Huige, 1977) have argued that it is important to distinguish "normal" (i.e., context- and situation-appropriate) dependence from "pathological" (i.e., maladaptive and inflexible) dependence, these researchers also concurred with the views of Neki (1976a), Ainsworth (1969), and Siegel (1988), noting that in general, dependency is associated with immaturity, weakness, and psychological impairment.

In this chapter, I trace the evolution of the dependency concept in psychology. I begin by providing an overview of the most important theoretical frameworks used by psychological researchers to derive and test hypotheses regarding the etiology and dynamics of dependent personality traits. I then discuss the different ways that developmental, clinical, and social psychologists have conceptualized and studied dependency. Finally, I offer a tentative "working definition" of dependency which can be tested against the results of relevant empirical studies that are described in subsequent chapters.

## THEORETICAL MODELS OF DEPENDENCY

Every theory of personality implicitly or explicitly includes a conceptual model of dependency. For example, humanistic personality theorists regard dependency primarily as a "defensive" behavior, the purpose of which is to minimize the anxiety and discomfort associated with an individual's failure to become fully self-actualized. In the humanistic perspective, the non-self-actualized person is hypothesized to be unwilling to engage in independent, self-directed behavior and instead relies on others for protection, guidance, and support (Maslow, 1970; Rogers, 1980).

Like humanistic personality theorists, existential theorists view dependency primarily as a defensive behavior (see Boss, 1977; May, 1969). To the existentialist, dependency represents an attempt to abrogate (i.e., externalize) responsibility for one's actions as a means of denying one's mortality and isolation in an unpredictable, uncontrollable world. Consequently, the dependent person's world view becomes increasingly narrowed and distorted. According to the existential model, dependent individuals ultimately come to regard themselves as (1) controlled by people and external events, (2) powerless to influence the outcome of events, and therefore (3) not responsible for the consequences of their behavior (Harrison, 1987).

Although every personality theory offers an associated theory of dependency, some theoretical perspectives have been more influential than others. Two models in particular have had a pervasive influence on dependency theory and research: the psychodynamic approach and the social learning view.

### The Psychodynamic Approach

In classical psychoanalytic theory, dependency is inextricably linked to the events of the infantile, "oral" stage of development (Freud, 1905/1953). Frustration or overgratification during the oral stage is hypothesized to result in oral "fixation" and an inability to resolve the developmental issues that characterize this stage (i.e., conflicts regarding dependence–independence). Thus, psychoanalytic theory postulates that the orally fixated (or "oral dependent") person will (1) remain dependent on others for nurturance and support and (2) continue to exhibit behaviors in adulthood that reflect the infantile oral stage (e.g., preoccupation with activities of the mouth, reliance on food and eating as a means of coping with anxiety).

Early in his career, Freud (1908/1953) discussed in general terms the links -between "fixation" and the development of particular personality traits, noting that "one very often meets with a type of character in which certain traits are very strongly marked while at the same time one's attention is arrested by the behavior of these persons in regard to certain bodily functions" (p. 167). Subsequently, Freud (1938/1964) was more explicit in linking personality development to the feeding experience during infancy, arguing that "a child sucking at his mother's breast becomes the prototype of every relation of love" (p. 222). The evolution of Freud's views on this topic paralleled what turned out to be, in retrospect, a pervasive trend in classical psychoanalytic theory, namely, an ever-increasing emphasis on social rather than biological factors as key elements in personality development.

Following Freud's (1905/1953, 1908/1955) initial speculations regarding the etiology and dynamics of oral dependency, several psychoanalytic writers (e.g., Abraham, 1927; Fenichel, 1945; Glover, 1925; Rado, 1928) extended the classical psychoanalytic model, suggesting that it was useful to distinguish two types of oral fixation: (1) oral fixation that resulted from frustration during infantile feeding and weaning and (2) oral fixation that resulted from overgratification during the feeding and weaning period. Infants who were overgratified during infancy were hypothesized to be overly optimistic. Thus, Abraham (1927) suggested that such individuals "have brought with them from this happy period a deeply rooted conviction that everything will always be well with them. They face life with an imperturbable optimism which often does in fact help them to achieve their aims" (p. 399). Goldman-Eisler (1948, 1950, 1951) subsequently elaborated on Abraham's hypotheses regarding the characteristics of "oral optimists," suggesting that in addition to being unrelentingly optimistic, such individuals were also likely to be sociable, nurturant, extroverted and ambitious.

In contrast, individuals whose oral dependency resulted from frustration during infancy were hypothesized to be overly pessimistic (Fenichel, 1945; Rado, 1928). Sandler and Dare (1970) provided a succinct summary of the classical psychoanalytic view regarding the traits, attitudes, and behaviors of these "oral pessimists," noting that "the orally frustrated or ungratified character has a characteristically pessimistic outlook on life which may be associated with moods of depression, attitudes of withdrawal, passive–receptive attitudes, feelings of insecurity with a need for constant reassurance . . . a dislike of sharing, and a general feeling of demanding coupled with dissatisfaction" (p. 216).[1]

There have been several attempts to test directly the hypotheses of Abraham (1927), Glover (1925), Fenichel (1945), and Rado (1928) regarding the division of oral dependent individuals into "oral optimists" and "oral pessimists" (Goldman-Eisler, 1948, 1950, 1951; Gottheil & Stone, 1968; Kline & Storey, 1977). Although some of these studies yielded promising findings (e.g., Goldman-Eisler, 1951), the majority of investigations in this area ultimately produced inconclusive results (see Kline & Storey [1977] and Masling & Schwartz [1979] for reviews of these studies).

During the past 20 years, psychoanalytic researchers have moved away from distinguishing subtypes of oral dependency, preferring to conceptualize oral dependency as a single personality dimension. The definition of oral dependency used by most researchers today is closer to that of the "oral pessimist" than that of the "oral optimist" (see Birtchnell, 1988a; Fisher & Greenberg, 1985; Masling, 1986; O'Neill & Bornstein, 1991).

Two subtle aspects of the classical psychoanalytic model warrant brief discussion at this point, because an awareness of these issues is key in understanding the logic that underlies researchers' approaches to operationalizing and testing the psychoanalytic model of oral dependency. First, it is important to keep in mind that although classical psychoanalytic theory argues that orally fixated persons are particularly preoccupied with unresolved infantile dependency needs, this model also suggests that everyone is to some extent preoccupied with these needs. In other words, the psychoanalytic model hypothesizes that everyone shows some degree of preoccupation with the developmental issues that characterize the infantile, oral stage. In psychoanalytic theory, oral fixation is conceptualized as a continuum, with those of us who are strongly orally fixated being more preoccupied with unresolved dependency needs than those of us who are less strongly fixated at the infantile, oral stage.

Second, it is important to keep in mind that in the classical psychoanalytic model, individuals are hypothesized to be unaware of their preoccupation with unresolved dependency needs. Clearly, it is unacceptable for adolescents and adults to express directly strong infantile dependency strivings. Thus, these needs are threatening and anxiety producing. Repression, denial, and other ego defenses act to keep the thoughts, wishes, and feelings associated with these infantile dependency needs out of awareness (see Parens & Saul, 1971; Silverman, Lachmann, & Milich, 1982). Although some adults may still have strong infantile dependency needs, these needs typically remain unconscious and are expressed indirectly (except for situations in which individuals become severely regressed, as can occur under conditions of severe stress, in certain forms of severe psychopathology such as schizophrenia) (see Silverman et al., 1982; Sperling & Berman, 1991).

Two theoretical models of dependency ultimately evolved from the classical psychoanalytic model: object relations theory and ethological (i.e., attachment) theory. Although object relations theory and attachment theory differ in some important ways, these two approaches also have much in common. Both models deemphasize the importance of actual "oral" activities (e.g., breastfeeding) in determining the development of oral dependent traits and behaviors (Greenberg & Mitchell, 1983). Instead, these models hypothesize that the overall quality of the infant–caretaker relationship during infancy and early childhood is the primary determinant of dependent traits in adulthood (Ainsworth, 1969; Blatt, 1974). In object relations theory and attachment theory, the infant's feeding and weaning experiences do not play a central role in determining later personality development. Rather, early feeding experiences are viewed as one aspect—albeit an important one—of the overall infant–caretaker relationship.

The object relations model of dependency extends the classical psychoanalytic model primarily by emphasizing separation–individuation and the emergence of the self-concept as critical developmental tasks that occur during infancy and early childhood. The most important implication of this conceptual shift—a shift that was already evident in certain of Freud's later writings (e.g., Freud, 1938/1964)—is that the infant–caretaker relationship is no longer viewed as being rooted exclusively in biological gratification provided by the caretaker to the infant. In object relations theory, social exchange between the infant and his or her caretaker replaces biological gratification provided by the caretaker as the key determinant of personality development. Self and object representations that are internalized (or introjected) during infancy and early childhood are hypothesized to play a central role in personality development and dynamics (Kernberg, 1976; Schafer, 1968). In this respect, object relations theory emphasizes the role of cognitive processes (e.g., mental representations and their related associative networks) as mediators of personality development and dynamics.

Object relations theory's emphasis on self and object representations as the building blocks of personality also represents an important conceptual shift away from the classical psychoanalytic view of oedipal dynamics as the key to personality development. By focusing on mental representations that are formed during infancy and early childhood, object relations theory alters the focus of psychoanalysis, shifting the theoretical emphasis from the study of oedipal dynamics to the phenomenon of infantile dependency as a causal factor in personality development and risk for psychopathology.

The ethological approach differs from the object relations model primarily in its emphasis on the innate, biological underpinnings of infant–mother bonding as a determinant of the self-concept and subsequent interpersonal behavior (Bowlby, 1969, 1973, 1980). In contrast to the object relations model, the ethological perspective combines concepts from psychoanalysis and evolutionary theory to account for individual differences in infant–caretaker bonding, and for the effects of these experiences on later personality development. In the ethological approach, the infant is seen as displaying increasingly complex and sophisticated attachment behaviors as physiological and cognitive maturation occurs. To some extent, individual differences in personality may be attributable to inherited predispositions, but equally important are the caretaker's responses to the infant's particular style of expressing attachment needs. Attachment theorists hypothesize that early infant–caretaker interactions result in the formation of internalized "working" models of self and others (Bowlby, 1980; Main, Kaplan, & Cassidy, 1985), which in turn influence the child's expectations regarding future interpersonal relationships.

In light of ethology's evolutionary roots, it is not surprising that infra-human research on attachment and bonding (e.g., Harlow, 1958) was initially an important impetus behind the development of the ethological approach. These early attachment studies helped to make explicit the complex ways in which the instinctual reactions and conditioned responses of infants and mothers interacted to produce infant–mother bonding in infra-humans. Only later were similar instinct-learning patterns identified in human infants and caretakers (see Ainsworth, 1969). In recent years, infrahuman attachment research has been increasingly influenced by ethological theories, so that the relationship between infrahuman research and ethology has become one of mutual influence and integration (Bowlby, 1980; Gewirtz, 1972).

## The Social Learning View

Early social learning models of dependency were strongly influenced by the work of drive theorists such as Hull (1943) and Mowrer (1950). Thus, it is not surprising that social learning theorists initially regarded dependency as an acquired drive, the impetus for which was the reduction of primary drives (e.g., hunger, anxiety) via the provision of primary reinforcers (e.g., food, warmth) within the context of the infant–caretaker relationship (see Dollard & Miller, 1950; Heathers, 1955a; Sears, 1972; Walters & Parke, 1964; Whiting, 1944). These early social learning models of dependency hypothesized that as the primary caretaker provides biological and psychological gratification to the infant (through feeding, providing warmth and contact comfort, etc.), she comes to be associated with pleasurable experiences and in effect becomes a kind of secondary reinforcer. To the extent that the infant's responses to the caretaker's protective, nurturing behavior generalize to other potential caretakers (e.g., teachers, supervisor, romantic partners), dependent behavior will continue to be exhibited in these relationships was well. Ainsworth (1969) provided a succinct summary of this "classical" social learning view, noting that in this model, dependency is regarded as "a class of behaviors, learned in the context of the infant's dependency relationship with his mother. . . .[A]lthough the first dependency relationship is a specific one, dependency is viewed as generalizing to subsequent interpersonal relationships" (p. 970).

Although some variants of social learning theory emphasize the importance of modeling as well as reinforcement in the development of dependent behaviors (see, e.g., Bandura, 1977; Bandura & Walters, 1963; Walters & Parke, 1964), social learning theories have in common the fundamental hypothesis that people *learn* to be dependent. Implicit in the social learning perspective is the assumption that dependent behaviors are exhibited because they are rewarded, were rewarded, or—at the very least—are perceived by the dependent person as likely to bring rewards. In short, this model hypothesizes that individual differences in adult dependency result from variations in the degree to which passive, dependent behavior was reinforced by the primary caretaker—and by other significant figures (e.g., siblings, teachers)—during early and middle childhood.

In at least one important respect, the evolution of the social learning model of dependency paralleled the evolution of the psychoanalytic view. Following early work in this area, theoreticians and researchers hypothesized that dependent individuals could be classified into two distinct subtypes. Although there were several notable efforts in this area, the most influential "independent subtype" social learning model of dependency was originally described by Heathers (1955a), who hypothesized that there are two independent dimensions of dependency—instrumental and emotional—which have different antecedents, correlates, and consequences. In Heathers's scheme, an individual may be "instrumentally dependent," "emotionally dependent," both, or neither.

Instrumental and emotional dependency differ in a number of ways (see Hartup, 1973; Marcus, 1976). However, the most useful distinction between these two constructs involves the goals of the child's attention-seeking behaviors. In this context, Heathers (1955a) suggested:

> [I]nstrumental dependence is present when a person seeks help in reaching goals. . . . When a child seeks help, as in getting food, help is the sub-goal in relation to the end-goal of food. With emotional dependence, the responses of others are the end-goals rather than the means of reaching them. The need for affection is an emotional-dependence need which is satisfied by others' affectionate responses. (p. 277)

In effect, Heathers argued that in instrumental dependency, other people's responses serve primarily as tools that help the child to obtain primary reinforcers, while in emotional dependency, other people's responses act as reinforcers in and of themselves.

Heathers's (1955a) model was quite influential during the late 1950s and early 1960s (Hartup, 1963; Walters & Parke, 1964). However, Heathers's conceptualization of dependency as consisting of separate "instrumentally dependent" and "emotionally dependent" subtypes was eventually sharply criticized (see, e.g., Gewirtz, 1972). Ultimately, this model was contradicted by a number of empirical findings. Most important, researchers were unable to demonstrate the existence of separate "instrumental" and "emotional" subtypes of the dependent personality. Rather, the behaviors that Heathers suggested would distinguish instrumental from emotional dependency actually showed moderate to strong intercorrelations in both children and adults (Beller, 1959; Hayakawa, 1977; Jamison & Comrey, 1968; Kagan & Moss, 1960; Livesley, Schroeder, & Jackson, 1990; Maccoby & Masters, 1970; Walters & Parke, 1964; Yeger & Miezitis, 1985).

Kagan and Moss's (1960) findings illustrate the general pattern of results obtained in studies of instrumental and emotional dependency. In Kagan and Moss's study, dependent behavior in a mixed-sex sample of 54 6–10-year-old children was assessed via a combination of parent ratings, experimenter ratings, ratings of classroom behavior, and in-home observations of parent–child interactions. Significant positive correlations between instrumental dependency scores and emotional dependency scores were found in both boys ($r = .60$) and girls ($r = .79$).

By the early 1970s, social learning researchers had moved beyond Heathers's (1955a) "independent subtype" conceptualization of dependency. With the advent of the cognitive revolution in psychology, social learning theorists increasingly emphasized the role of cognitive processes (rather than conditioned responses) as mediators of passive and dependent traits and behaviors (Abramson, Seligman, & Teasdale, 1978; Bandura, 1977; Mischel, 1970, 1973; Mischel & Peake, 1982). As the emphasis in social learning theory shifted from conditioned responses to cognitive processes, dependency became increasingly linked with depression. In fact, many social learning theorists now view dependency primarily in terms of a cognitive (or attributional) "style" in which an individual perceives him- or herself as powerless, helpless, and unable to influence the outcome of events in a positive way. Distortions in the processing of information regarding causes (and effects) of positive and negative events propagate the dependent person's belief in his or her own ineffectiveness, reinforce the idea that he or she needs to rely on others for guidance and support, and may lead to increased risk for certain forms of depression (Abramson et al., 1978).

Without question, the cognitive revolution changed social learning theory in fundamental ways. However, another important conceptual shift in social learning theory and research also occurred in the late 1960s and early 1970s—a shift that was completely independent of the cognitive revolution. Although social learning theorists had long been interested in the effects of sex-role socialization on the overt expression of dependency needs (see, e.g., Sears, Maccoby, & Levin, 1957; Sears, Whiting, Nowlis, & Sears, 1953), sex-role socialization research moved from the periphery to the mainstream of social learning theory in the early 1970s. This was due primarily to researchers' increasing awareness of the powerful and pervasive effects of sex-role socialization on personality development (Maccoby & Jacklin, 1974; Spence & Helmreich, 1978), on the development of the self-concept (Singh, 1981; White, 1986), and on cultural norms regarding political, social, and economic power and influence (McClain, 1978; Siegel, 1988; Symour, 1977).

Clearly, sex-role socialization influences men's and women's dependency needs and dependent behaviors in a number of ways. Typically, traditional sex-role socialization practices discourage men from expressing openly dependent feelings, thoughts, and behaviors. In contrast, traditional sex-role socialization practices encourage women to express their dependency needs openly, because overt dependent behavior is consistent with the traditional female sex role. Lytton and Romney (1991) provided an excellent review and meta-analysis of research on gender differences in sex-role socialization practices. Their findings make explicit what most of us already suspect, namely, that dependent behavior is more strongly discouraged in boys than in girls. This pattern of gender differences in sex-role socialization is consistent across different cultures, across different subcultures within American society, and across different ethnic groups and social classes.[2]

Of course, parents are not solely responsible for the differential socialization of boys and girls with respect to the overt expression of underlying dependency needs. There is ample evidence that teachers, older siblings, and other role models (e.g., fictional heroes and heroines) (see White, 1986) also encourage children—either subtly or directly—to conform to traditional sex-role expectations (Spence & Helmreich, 1978). Furthermore, observational learning appears to play a key role in the development of sex-typed behaviors, including the overt expression of dependency needs (Mischel, 1970). In this respect, media figures may also influence the degree to which dependency needs are expressed openly in men and women.

Needless to say, although men are discouraged from expressing dependency needs openly, men's dependency needs do not simply disappear. Rather, they can be either expressed indirectly or not expressed at all. The same is true of women's *independency* (i.e., autonomy) needs. Several writers have commented on the ways in which men's dependency needs and women's needs for autonomy and independence are expressed indirectly within friendships and romantic relationships (e.g., Baumrind, 1980; Gilbert, 1987; Kaplan, 1983; Lerner, 1983; Pleck, 1981). The fact remains, however, that because traditional sex-role socialization practices discourage men from expressing dependency needs openly, and discourage women from expressing independency needs openly, these socialization practices create conflict and ambivalence regarding dependency in both men and women, as each of us is taught to relinquish a fundamental group of "gender-inappropriate" needs. In this context, Lerner (1983) suggested that "the struggle to achieve a healthy integration of passive–dependent longings and active autonomous strivings consitutes a life-long developmental task for both men and women" (p. 697).

# THE PSYCHOANALYTIC AND SOCIAL LEARNING MODELS OF DEPENDENCY: A COMPARISON

At first glance, the psychoanalytic and social learning models of dependency appear to have little in common. Nothing could be further from the truth. To be sure, there is at least one fundamental difference between these two theoretical perspectives: Psychoanalytic theory hypothesizes that the dependent person will be preoccupied with "oral" activities (e.g., eating, drinking, smoking), whereas the social learning model makes no prediction regarding a link between dependency and these behaviors. In operational terms, this hypothesis translates into two more specific predictions. First, as discussed earlier, psychoanalytic theory hypothesizes that the etiology of dependency lies in infantile feeding and weaning activities. Second, psychoanalytic theory hypothesizes that level of dependency should predict the likelihood of cigarette smoking, risk for alcoholism, and risk for obesity and other eating disorders (e.g., anorexia). These hypotheses turn out to be very important, because they allow the predictive validity of the psychoanalytic and social learning models to be compared directly via an analysis of relevant empirical findings (see Chapters 3 and 6 for detailed comparisons of the psychoanalytic and social learning models with respect to these two hypotheses).

Aside from these differences between the psychoanalytic and social learning models, there are a number of important similarities between these two theoretical perspectives. Although psychoanalysis and social learning theory use different language to describe certain ideas, careful examination of these ideas reveals that they actually have much in common. In the following sections, I briefly describe three areas in which psychoanalysis and social learning theory describe parallel concepts in slightly different ways.

## Dependency Conflict

Both the psychoanalytic and social learning models predict that individuals will be conflicted (i.e., strongly ambivalent) regarding underlying dependency needs. However, the roots of this conflict differ in the two models. In psychoanalysis, infantile dependency needs are hypothesized to be almost completely unconscious in adults. Ego defenses (e.g., repression, denial, reaction formation) prevent these needs from being experienced directly. In addition, individuals may use conscious countercontrol strategies (e.g., deliberate suppression of dependent thoughts and feelings) to avoid expressing dependency needs that become conscious. Thus, dependency conflict within the psychoanalytic model is conceptualized as a struggle between unconscious dependency needs and conscious prohibitions against expressing these needs.

In social learning theory, dependency conflict arises from inconsistent socialization practices that almost inevitably occur during early and middle childhood. On the one hand, children are taught to obey figures of authority (e.g., parents, teachers), to depend on figures of authority for nurturance, protection, and guidance, and to value social reinforcements offered by authority figures (e.g., compliments, grades). On the other hand, children—especially boys—are taught to be creative, autonomous, and independent in work and in play. In other words, children are socialized to believe that there are important rewards to be obtained by being dependent and important rewards to be obtained by being independent. Conflict is created as the child attempts to resolve these two conflicting messages and to determine which type of behavior—dependent or independent—is appropriate in a particular situation.

## The Social Roots of Dependency

Both psychoanalytic theory and social learning theory emphasize the social roots of dependency, although they do so in different ways. In psychoanalysis, dependency originates in the infant–caretaker dyad, that is, in the infant's first social relationship. As noted earlier, this first relationship is hypothesized to serve as a prototype for later interpersonal relationships. In social learning theory, dependency also originates in the infant–caretaker dyad, for it is within this relationship that early socialization takes place. However, in contrast to psychoanalytic theory, social learning theory hypothesizes that later social relationships—both within and outside the family—contribute in important ways to the child's beliefs and expectations regarding dependency.

## Cognitive Processes Underlying Dependency

In psychoanalytic theory, mental representations of the parents and other significant figures play a key role in determining the degree to which a person experiences (and expresses) strong dependency needs. In social learning theory, beliefs and expectations regarding rewards and punishments associated with expressing dependency needs openly play a key role in determining a person's dependency-related behaviors. Clearly, mental representations are not the same thing as beliefs and expectations. However, the creation of internalized mental representations and the acquisition of beliefs regarding acceptable interpersonal behaviors have one important thing in common: Both are, above all, cognitive processes that involve the construction of abstract categories representing conceptually and functionally similar stimuli and events, and the ability to apply (i.e., generalize) past experiences to novel situations.

## DOMAINS OF DEPENDENCY RESEARCH

Ironically, although there has been an increasing emphasis on cognitive processes as mediators of dependent traits and behaviors, both in object relations theory and in the social learning model, there have been few studies examining the cognitive correlates of dependency. To be sure, many studies of dependency involve the assessment of attitudes, interpersonal perceptions, and beliefs regarding the self and others (see Fisher & Greenberg, 1985; Masling, 1986). Other studies have examined the relationship of dependency to cognitive style and creativity (e.g., Holt, 1966). However, in most of these investigations cognitive processes are assessed only as a means to an end. In other words, dependency researchers utilize cognitive constructs primarily as a tool to test basic hypotheses regarding the etiology, dynamics, and correlates of dependency. Virtually all dependency research conducted to date has come from three domains within psychology: developmental, clinical, and social. In the following sections, I describe the evolution of the dependency concept in these three domains.

## Developmental

To the developmental psychologist, dependency represents a normal developmental phase through which all individuals progress (albeit to different degrees and at different rates) as maturation occurs. In this respect, childhood dependency is ubiquitous, and hence, unremarkable. However, developmental researchers have also examined individual differences in childhood and adolescent dependency. Much of this research has focused on the antecedents and correlates of exaggerated dependency needs in children and adolescents, and on the effects of exaggerated dependency needs on social and personality development (Kaul, Mathur, & Murlidharan, 1982).

In developmental psychology, dependency has historically been linked with attachment behavior during infancy and early childhood (Ainsworth, 1969, 1972) and with the emergence of the self-concept (Mahler, Pine, & Bergman, 1975). Although there is some overlap between the constructs of dependency and attachment as most researchers define them, these constructs are not one and the same (see Feeney & Noller, 1990; Gewirtz, 1972; Kaul et al., 1982; West, Livesley, Reiffer, & Sheldon, 1986). Clearly, dependency is an important component of certain forms of attachment behavior (e.g., insecure attachment), both in childhood (Sroufe, 1983; Sroufe, Fox, & Pancake, 1983; Waters & Deane, 1985) and during adolescence and adulthood (Blatt & Homann, 1992; Hendrick & Hendrick, 1989; Sperling & Berman, 1991). However, individual differences in attachment and dependency in children have different antecedents (Sroufe et al., 1983) and correlates (Ainsworth, 1969), and predict different aspects of adult behavior (Kaul et al., 1982; Livesley et al., 1990). Furthermore, the behaviors that characterize dependency and insecure attachment show only moderate overlap, both conceptually (Ainsworth, 1969, 1972; Maccoby & Masters, 1970; Waters & Deane, 1985) and empirically (Heathers, 1955b; Sears, Rau, & Alpert, 1965; Sroufe et al., 1983; Turner, 1991; West et al., 1986).

Not surprisingly, developmental researchers' operational definitions of dependency and attachment differ substantially (see Cairns, 1972; Sears, 1972; West et al., 1986). As Livesley et al. (1990) noted, attachment behavior typically refers to

> any form of behavior that results in a person attaining or retaining proximity to some preferred individual, who is usually conceived as stronger and/or wiser. Dependency behaviors, in contrast, are not directed toward a specific individual, nor are they concerned with promoting the feelings of security that arise from proximity to attachment figures. Instead, they are more generalized behaviors designed to elicit assistance, guidance and approval [from others]. (p. 132)

Similarly, Ainsworth (1972) argued that "attachment is an affectional tie or bond that one individual (person or animal) forms between himself and another specific individual. In contrast, dependency is a generalized or nonfocused response characteristic" (p. 100). In short, attachment behavior is manifested primarily by proximity seeking, while dependent behavior is manifested primarily by help seeking. Moreover, attachment behaviors are "object specific" and are consistently directed toward the same person. In contrast, dependent behaviors may be directed toward any number of people who represent, in the eyes of the dependent person, potential nurturers, protectors, or caretakers.[3]

Recent research on attachment in adolescents and adults is consistent with a conceptualization of attachment as involving specific proximity-seeking behaviors directed at a single individual (as opposed to the more generalized help-seeking stance typically associated with dependency) (see Ainsworth, 1989; Collins & Read, 1990; Feeney & Noller, 1990; Hazan & Shaver, 1987; Simpson, 1990; Sperling & Berman, 1991). Unfortunately, however, the links between dependency and attachment in adolescents and adults remain largely unexplored, and the degree to which adolescents and adults who show an "insecure" attachment style also show exaggerated dependency needs (e.g., help seeking, need for guidance and approval from others) remains open to question.

Until the early 1980s, developmental psychologists focused almost exclusively on the antecedents, correlates, and consequences of childhood dependency. However, in recent years developmental psychologists have begun to examine dependency in older adults as well (see, e.g., Barton,

Baltes, & Orzech, 1980; Beall & Goldstein, 1982). This increasing attention to dependency in older adults reflects researchers' general interest in creating theories of development that account for changes in personality and social interaction across the entire lifespan. To date, developmental research on dependency in the elderly has tended to focus on overall changes in dependency levels that occur from middle to late adulthood (see Helson & Wink, 1992). However, as interest in the correlates and consequences of dependency in older adults continues to grow, it is likely that researchers will begin to examine individual differences in dependency in the elderly, as they now do in children, adolescents, and younger adults.

## Clinical

Early clinical descriptions of individuals with exaggerated dependency needs were quite negative. For example, Kraeplin (1913) characterized the dependent individual as "shiftless," while Schneider (1923) referred to dependent persons as "weak willed." This negative view was propagated by early psychoanalytic theorists (Abraham, 1927; Fenichel, 1945; Freud, 1938/1964), and by various neoanalytic theorists (Fromm, 1947; Horney, 1945; Sullivan, 1947). Fromm (1947) provided one of the more articulate early descriptions of the dependent personality, noting that these individuals

> are dependent not only on authorities for knowledge and help, but on people in general for any kind of support. They feel lost when alone because they feel that they cannot do anything without help. It is characteristic of these people that their first thought is to find somebody else to give them needed information rather than to make even the slightest effort on their own. (p. 62)

Abraham's (1927) and Fenichel's (1945) descriptions of "oral dependent" individuals are very similar to Fromm's (1947) view of "receptive" persons.

Several dependency-related issues have received substantial attention from clinicians and clinical researchers. For example, numerous clinicians have explored the impact of patient dependency on the psychotherapeutic process. It is clear that dependency is an inescapable aspect of the therapeutic relationship, and that dependency issues frequently arise during insight-oriented psychotherapy (Colgan, 1987; Gilbert, 1987; Lerner, 1983; Neki, 1976b). Moreover, therapists agree that when dependency issues become prominent in therapy, they can play a central role in transference (and countertransference) dynamics (see Emery & Lesher, 1982; Hopkins, 1986; Pakes, 1975; Ryder & Parry-Jones, 1982; Snyder, 1963). However, therapists do not agree regarding whether, overall, patient dependency helps or hinders the psychotherapeutic process. On the one hand, Dollard and Miller (1950) suggested that patient dependency can facilitate psychotherapy insofar as dependency needs motivate the patient to perform well in therapy in order to please the therapist. On the other hand, dependency can become a problem in psychotherapy (and in medical treatment as well), if the patient's dependency needs cause her to cling to the patient role and resist relinquishing the doctor–patient relationship as termination or discharge nears (Rogers, 1942).

Balint (1964) summarized nicely the ambivalent attitude that many psychotherapists have regarding patient dependency. He noted:

> [T]here are many factors in every doctor-patient relationship which push the patient into a dependent, childish relationship to his doctor. This is inevitable. The only question is how much dependence is desirable . . . how much dependence consitutes a good starting point for successful therapy, and when does it turn into an obstacle. (pp. 39–40)

In this context, some researchers have suggested that psychotherapy will be facilitated if the therapist does not interfere with a dependent transference relationship early in therapy, but increasingly discourages the patient from exhibiting dependent, help-seeking behaviors as therapy progresses (Crowder, 1972).

Along different lines, numerous theoreticians and clinical researchers have suggested that dependency may be a risk factor for certain psychological disorders. Early speculation in this area focused primarily on the hypothesized links between dependency and depression, although psychoanalytically oriented clinicians and researchers also discussed the possible role of dependency as a risk factor for alcoholism and other disorders that appeared to have a clear connection with "orality" and "oral fixation" (e.g., smoking, eating disorders) (see Greenberg & Bornstein, 1988b). Social learning theorists subsequently extended the concept of dependency as a risk factor for psychopathology to other areas, suggesting that a variety of psychological disorders—not only those with an obvious "oral" component—may be linked to exaggerated dependency needs (see, e.g., Bandura, 1977).

Finally, clinical researchers have conceptualized exaggerated dependency needs as a form of psychopathology in and of itself. This view has been formalized in the diagnostic category of Dependent Personality Disorder (DPD), which appears in both the DSM-III (American Psychological Association [APA], 1980) and DSM-III-R (APA, 1987). As is true of the other Axis II personality disorders described in the DSM-III and DSM-III-R, DPD is regarded primarily as a dysfunctional interpersonal style that is associated with (1) a pattern of maladaptive and/or self-destructive behaviors and (2) increased risk for certain psychological disorders (Millon, 1981).

Needless to say, clinicians and clinical researchers continue to show strong interest in the dynamics of dependency, and numerous anecdotal

descriptions of the dependent personality have been offered. These anecdotal accounts are far too numerous to describe or classify here. However,
two recent descriptions warrant attention because (1) they reflect the general tone of most clinicians' descriptions of the dependent individual and (2)
they illustrate how little change has occurred in clinicians' perceptions of
dependency during the past 50 years. Thus, Millon (1981) argued:

> [D]ependent persons' "centers of gravity" lie in others, not in themselves.
> They adapt their behavior to please those on whom they depend. . . . Depen-
> dent personalities tend to denigrate themselves and their accomplishments.
> What self-esteem they possess is determined largely by the support and en-
> couragement of others. . . . To protect themselves, dependents quickly submit
> and comply with what others wish, or make themselves so pleasing that no one
> could possibly want to abandon them. (p. 107)

Birtchnell's (1988a) description of the dependent person parallels
Millon's (1981) view. Birtchnell (1988a) described the dependent person
as having "the need to stay close to others, the inclination to be primarily
the recipient in interpersonal transactions, and the tendency to relate to
others from a position of inferiority and humility" (p. 111). Similar descriptions of dependency may be found in Carnes (1984), Fisher and
Greenberg (1985), Masling (1986), and Parens and Saul (1971). These
descriptions are virtually indistinguishable from those offered by Fenichel
(1945), Fromm (1947), Horney (1945), and Sullivan (1947) nearly 50
years ago.

## Social

Social psychologists have had an ambivalent relationship with the concept
of dependency. During the past several decades, social researchers have
conducted numerous studies examining the relationship of dependency to
interpersonal perceptions, beliefs, and behaviors. However, although dependency is clearly a topic of considerable interest to social psychologists,
dependency research has not yet made its way into mainstream social psychology. It remains on the sidelines, never having received the kind of
in-depth discussion and integration into the core of the discipline that other
widely studied individual difference variables (e.g., authoritarianism, need
for affiliation, self-monitoring) have received. This is particularly ironic
because dependency is, by definition, a trait that is manifested primarily in
interpersonal (i.e., social) interactions.

Social research on dependency can be divided into two domains. Beginning with Thibaut and Kelley's (1959) classic analysis of interpersonal
transactions within groups, numerous researchers have examined the effects
of "social dependence" on individuals' social perceptions and behaviors (see

Strong, Welsh, Corcoran, & Hoyt [1992] for a review of research in this area). As Strong et al. (1992) noted, social dependence has traditionally been defined as a situation wherein "[another] person possesses or controls resources, and . . . the person himself or herself is experiencing needs related to the resources" (p. 147). Although Thibaut and Kelley's concept of social dependence focuses primarily on situational variables that create a power differential between two individuals, the parallels between situationally induced social dependence and individual differences in trait dependency are easy to see.

The prevailing social view of dependency as an individual difference variable can be traced to Murray's (1938) discussion of "basic needs," certain of which (e.g., need for succorance, need for nurturance) simultaneously reflect social motivations and dependency-related traits and behaviors. In this context, Walters and Parke (1964) suggested that for social researchers, the term "dependency" has been used

> both as a behavioral and as a motivational construct . . . it has referred to a set of interrelated and presumably substitutable responses such as asking for help or reassurance, seeking physical contact, and attracting the attention of others. Such responses have been regarded as sharing the characteristic of being capable of eliciting attending and ministering responses from others, or of being instrumental in obtaining social reinforcement. (pp. 239–240)

Studies by Schachter (1959) and others (e.g., Crowne & Marlowe, 1964) that were derived in part from this theoretical framework played a significant role in stimulating social psychologists' early interest in dependency. More recently, social researchers have begun to examine the cognitive and attributional correlates of dependency, bringing dependency research into line with models of social information processing that have come to dominate present-day social psychology.

Social psychologists, like clinical psychologists, tend to view dependency primarily in negative terms (see Assor, Aronoff, & Messe, 1981; Walters & Parke, 1964). However, the social view of dependency is not nearly as negative as the clinical view. On the one hand, Assor et al. (1981) describe the dependent person as "interested primarily in avoiding responsibility and interpersonal conflict; they try to compensate for their sense of helplessness by obtaining the support of others through occupying a lower status or follower position" (p. 790). Bales (1970), Leary (1957), and others have similarly emphasized the passive qualities of dependent individuals and the tendency of dependent persons to subjugate themselves and their needs in order to please others.

However, other social researchers have focused on more positive aspects of dependency. For example, Banu and Puhan (1983) suggested that because dependent persons are concerned with being supported and helped by others, they should have empathy for individuals in need and should be particularly likely to assist a person in trouble. Along different lines, a number of researchers (e.g., Baker & Reitz, 1978; Berkowitz & Daniels, 1963, 1964; Taylor, Messick, Lehman, & Hirsch, 1982) have argued that dependency can serve as a social cue that, under certain circumstances, causes other people to work harder because they conclude that the dependent person is helpless and unable to fend for him- or herself. Finally, some researchers (e.g., Battistich & Aronoff, 1985) maintain that in certain situations, dependent individuals may be perceived more favorably by others than are nondependent persons.

## DEFINING DEPENDENCY

In light of the fact that dependency research has taken place in three different domains and has drawn on at least two different theoretical frameworks, it is not surprising that psychologists have been unable to formulate a universally accepted operational definition of dependency. Some researchers have been content to offer relatively loose, descriptive definitions of dependency (see Carnes, 1984; Hirschfeld et al., 1977; Parens & Saul, 1971; Sinha, 1968; Wilkin, 1987). For example, Hirschfeld et al. (1977) describe dependency as "a complex of thoughts, beliefs, feelings and behaviors which revolve around the need to associate closely with, interact with, and rely upon valued other people" (p. 610). Sinha (1968) was even more succinct (albeit somewhat tautological), in his definition of dependency as "a motivational habit of overdependence on others in situations in which dependence is not really called for" (p. 66).

Other researchers have taken a more systematic approach to this issue, attempting to delineate the various subtraits that compose the dependent personality in children and adults (e.g., Beller, 1955, 1957; Birtchnell, 1984, 1987, 1988a, 1991b; Finney, 1965, 1966; Gewirtz, 1956a; Goldman-Eisler, 1948, 1951; Gottheil, 1965a, 1965b; Jamison & Comrey, 1968; Kline & Storey, 1977, 1980; Lazare, Klerman, & Armor, 1966, 1970; Novy, 1992; Pilkonis, 1988; Sears, 1972). Correlational and factor-analytic studies conducted by these (and other) researchers confirm that dependency is in fact composed of a number of theoretically related subtraits, including self-reports of passivity, suggestibility, interpersonal compliance, conflict–avoidance, pessimism, self-doubt, emotional reliance on others, lack of social self-confidence, conformity, help seeking and need for approval.

In lieu of a specific operational definition of dependency, I offer a tentative "working definition" of this construct that can be tested against the results of relevant empirical studies. I propose that dependency is a personality style (or "type") that is characterized by four primary components: (1) *motivational* (i.e., a marked need for guidance, approval, and support from others); (2) *cognitive* (i.e., a perception of the self as relatively powerless and ineffectual, along with the belief that others are powerful and can control the outcome of situations); (3) *affective* (i.e., a tendency to become anxious and fearful when required to function independently, especially when the products of one's efforts are to be evaluated by others); and (4) *behavioral* (i.e., a tendency to seek help, support, approval, guidance, and reassurance from others and to yield to others in interpersonal transactions).

## NOTES

1. A slightly different approach to this issue was discussed by Abraham (1927), who suggested that it was useful to distinguish "oral dependent" from "oral aggressive" personalities, the former characterized primarily by passivity and helplessness and the latter characterized by aggressiveness and intrusiveness. There is considerable overlap between Abraham's dependent–aggressive distinction and the frustration–overgratification distinction proposed by Glover (1925) and others. Most researchers have preferred to utilize the frustration–overgratfication distinction in lieu of the dependent–aggressive dichotomy (see Sandler & Dare, 1970).

2. Although Lytton and Romney's (1991) results indicated that there is substantial cross-cultural consistency in parents' differential socialization of boys and girls with respect to the overt expression of dependency needs, one limitation of these results warrants mention. Lytton and Romney included in their review only studies that involved subjects from Western countries (e.g., America, Canada, Mexico, Great Britain, Ireland). However, evidence suggests that the socialization patterns typically found in Western societies may not be characteristic of certain non-Western societies. In particular, it seems that socialization practices regarding the expression of dependency needs are quite different in Japan (Doi, 1973; Kobayashi, 1989) and India (Neki, 1976a; Sinha, 1968) than they are in most other cultures. In Japan and India, both boys and girls have historically been encouraged to express dependency needs openly (see also Bloom [1982], Danzinger [1960], and Parker [1960] for examples of other dependency-related socialization practices in non-Western societies).

3. I do not mean to imply by this discussion that dependency and attachment are completely unrelated. Clearly, children who show an insecure attachment style also tend to show exaggerated dependent behaviors (Sroufe, 1983). Moreover, certain qualities of the infant–caretaker relationship that result in the development of an insecure attachment style also produce high levels of dependency during middle and late childhood (see Ainsworth, 1972; Maccoby & Masters, 1970), and it may well be that insecure attachment is a precursor of dependency in many children. In fact, even in adulthood, insecure attachment is associated with high

levels of interpersonal dependency (Bartholomew & Horowitz, 1991). Without question, the relationship between dependency and attachment is complex, and warrants continued attention from developmental researchers. Nonetheless, I believe that, consistent with the suggestions of Ainsworth (1969, 1972), Sears (1972) and others, attachment and dependency are best conceptualized as distinct and different—albeit related—concepts.

# Assessing Dependency

Because the concept of dependency is of interest to researchers in a wide variety of areas, numerous measures of dependency have been developed. A thorough review of the empirical literature reveals that researchers have constructed and validated more than 35 separate dependency measures since the late 1940s. Although some of these measures are quite obscure and have been used only rarely, others have stood the test of time and continue to be widely used by developmental, social, and clinical researchers. Among the more widely used dependency measures are Navran's (1954) Minnesota Mulitphasic Personality Inventory (MMPI) dependency (Dy) scale; Masling, Rabie, and Blondheim's (1967) Rorschach Oral Dependency (ROD) scale; Sinha's (1968) Dependence Proneness (DP) scale; the dependency subscale of Blatt, D'Afflitti, and Quinlan's (1976) Depressive Experiences Questionnaire (DEQ); a factor-analytically derived Measure of Interpersonal Dependency (MID) (Hirschfeld et al., 1977); the Blacky test oral dependency scale (Blum, 1949); the Lazare–Klerman (LK) oral dependency scale (Lazare et al., 1966, 1970); the Holtzman Inkblot Test (HIT) dependency scale (Fisher, 1970); the Millon Clinical Multiaxial Inventory (MCMI) Dependency scale (Millon, 1987); Beck, Epstein, Harrison, and Emery's (1983) Sociotropy–Autonomy Scale (SAS); TAT-derived dependency scales (Kagan & Mussen, 1956); and combinations of subscales from Edwards's (1959) Personal Preference Schedule (EPPS). In addition, in the clinical setting researchers have used DSM-III (APA, 1980) or DSM-III-R (APA, 1987) criteria for DPD to select dependent subjects for study.

There are also a number of dependency scales that—for one reason or another—tend to be less widely used than are the dependency measures just listed. These scales fall into four categories. First, researchers have occasionally utilized projective measures such as sentence completion tests, the Hand Test (Wagner, 1983), or frequency counts of "spontaneous" oral dependent associations to assess dependency (see Fisher [1970], Lenihan & Kirk [1990], O'Neill, Greenberg, & Fisher [1984], and Sinha [1968] for examples of studies using these measures). Second, some investigators have used behavioral (i.e., observational) measures of dependency (Moskowitz, 1982; Smith & Bain, 1978; Watson, 1957); peer, parent, or teacher ratings (Fitzgerald, 1958; Kagan & Moss, 1960; Wiggins & Winder, 1961; Zuckerman, 1958); or interview ratings (Becker, Peterson, Luria, Shoemaker, & Hellmer, 1962; Zuckerman, Levitt, & Lubin, 1961). Third, researchers have occasionally utilized Q-sort techniques to assess level of dependency in children and adults (see, e.g., Block, 1971; Caspi, Bem, & Elder, 1989). Finally, a few researchers have utilized self-report measures of dependency specifically designed for use in a particular study (e.g., Berscheid & Fei, 1977; Birtchnell, 1988b; Lapan & Patton, 1986; Rossman, 1984; Schlenker & Weigold, 1990; Tesser & Blusiewicz, 1987).

In this chapter, I provide a brief overview of the various dependency measures used by developmental, clinical, and social researchers. I first discuss objective and projective measures of dependency. Next, I describe various rating and interview procedures that have been used to identify dependent individuals. Finally, I review research that examines the psychometric properties of these dependency measures.

## OBJECTIVE AND PROJECTIVE
## DEPENDENCY MEASURES

The 12 most widely used objective and projective dependency scales are listed in Table 2.1. This table also lists the "source" of each scale (i.e., the paper in which the scale was first described and/or employed) and provides information regarding the content and structure of each measure. As Table 2.1 shows, these 12 dependency measures can be classified along two dimensions: content (i.e., measures of "interpersonal dependency" versus measures of "oral dependency") and format (i.e., objective versus projective). Thus, there are four general types of dependency scales: objective interpersonal, objective oral, projective interpersonal and projective oral. Perusal of Table 2.1 reveals that the most widely used dependency measures are not equally distributed across these four categories. Of the 12 dependency measures listed in this table, 7 are objective interpersonal scales, 1 is a projective interpersonal scale, 3 are projective oral measures, and 1 is an objective oral measure.

Clearly, there is a tendency for interpersonal dependency scales to utilize an objective format, and for oral dependency scales to use a projective format. This pattern is not surprising, given that (1) oral dependency measures are invariably tied to psychoanalytic theory and (2) historically, psychoanalytic researchers have been more favorably disposed toward projective measures than have nonpsychoanalytic researchers (see Lindzey, 1959; Lubin, Larsen, & Matarazzo, 1984). A statistical analysis of the

**TABLE 2.1. Frequently Used Objective and Projective Dependency Scales**

| Scale | Source | Type of scale | |
| | | Content | Structure |
| --- | --- | --- | --- |
| Blacky test oral dependency scale | Blum (1949) | Or | Pro |
| MMPI Dy scale | Navran (1954) | Int | Obj |
| TAT dependency scale | Kagan & Mussen (1956) | Int | Pro |
| EPPS | Edwards (1959) | Int | Obj |
| LK oral dependency scale | Lazare et al. (1966) | Or | Obj |
| ROD scale | Masling et al. (1967) | Or | Pro |
| DP scale | Sinha (1968) | Int | Obj |
| HIT dependency scale | Fisher (1970) | Or | Pro |
| DEQ dependency scale | Blatt et al. (1976) | Int | Obj |
| MID | Hirschfeld et al. (1977) | Int | Obj |
| SAS | Beck et al. (1983) | Int | Obj |
| MCMI dependency scale | Millon (1987) | Int | Obj |

*Note.* For content, Or = oral dependency; Int = interpersonal dependency. For structure, Obj = objective test; Pro = projective test.

distribution of the two types of dependency scale contents across the two types of dependency scale formats confirms what perusal of Table 2.1 suggests, namely, that this distribution is not random ($\chi^2$ [1, $n = 12$] = 4.69, $p < .03$).

Because the dependency scales listed in Table 2.1 have been used so frequently during the past several decades, it is worth discussing these scales in a bit more detail. In the following sections, I briefly describe the four types of dependency measures that comprise the 12 scales listed in Table 2.1.

## Objective Measures

In general, objective interpersonal dependency measures require subjects to respond to direct questions regarding dependent thoughts, feelings, and behaviors. Typically, test items in these scales consist of a series of self-statements. The majority of objective interpersonal dependency measures employ a true–false format (e.g., the MID and MMPI Dy scale), although a few of these measures require subjects to make Likert-type ratings (e.g., 5- or 7-point ratings) of the degree to which statements in particular test items apply to them (e.g., the DP scale and DEQ dependency scale). In general, objective interpersonal dependency measures have high face validity (i.e., are obviously tapping dependency-related traits). For example, items on Hirschfeld et al.'s (1977) MID include the following: "When I have a decision to make, I always ask for advice," and "I am quick to agree with the opinions expressed by others." Similarly, Blatt et al.'s (1976) DEQ Dependency scale includes such items as "Without support from others who are close to me, I would be helpless" and "I find it very difficult to say no to the requests of friends." Typical statements on Sinha's (1968) DP scale are as follows: "Before making a serious decision, one should consult one's good friends or an experienced person," and "It is better to go along with the majority than to have one's own way."

Objective oral dependency measures utilize the same self-statement format as do objective interpersonal dependency measures. However, because objective oral dependency measures are closely tied to psychoanalytic theory, they require subjects to respond to questions regarding preoccupation with food, eating, and other "oral" activities in addition to questions regarding dependent thoughts, feelings, and behaviors. Thus, the LK oral dependency scale (Lazare et al., 1966, 1970) includes not only dependency-related items such as "I am easily swayed by others," but also such "oral" items as "When in a rage, I tend to physically express my feelings by grinding my teeth, pushing my hand into my mouth, biting my fingernails or handkerchief or other objects, or tearing something."

Objective dependency scales (both interpersonal and oral) typically yield several dependency-related subscale scores in addition to a global dependency score. In most cases, these subscales were derived via factor analysis or cluster analysis (see, e.g., Hirschfeld et al., 1977; Lazare et al., 1966, 1970; Sinha, 1968; Vandenberg & Helstone, 1975). Because objective dependency measures yield scores on separate dependency-related subscales, these measures can provide information regarding specific dependent attitudes, beliefs, and behaviors. This allows researchers to examine the interrelationship of various dependency-related subtraits and to assess the relationship of specific dependency-related subtraits to relevant outcome measures.

As might be expected, different objective dependency measures use somewhat different subscales. For example, the MID (Hirschfeld et al., 1977) yields three dependency-related subscale scores: (1) emotional reliance on others, (2) lack of social self-confidence, and (3) lack of autonomy. In contrast, the DP scale (Sinha, 1968) yields four dependency-related subscale scores: (1) help seeking, (2) lack of autonomy, (3) passivity, and (4) conformity/compliance. Along different lines, the LK oral dependency scale (Lazare et al., 1966, 1970) yields five subscale scores, four of which are related to dependent behavior and one of which is related to preoccupation with oral activities. The five subscales of the LK oral dependency scale are (1) dependence, (2) pessimism, (3) passivity, (4) acceptance/rejection of others, and (5) oral aggression.

## Projective Measures

Projective dependency measures require subjects to respond to ambiguous stimuli such as inkblots or drawings. Subjects' responses are then scored by the experimenter for either dependent content (as in the case of Kagan & Mussen's [1956] TAT dependency scale) or oral dependent content (as in the case of Masling et al.'s [1967] ROD scale). The ambiguity inherent in projective dependency measures represents an important strength: Because subjects are not aware of what information the experimenter plans to extract from their responses, projective dependency measures have low face validity and are relatively immune from self-report and self-presentation biases. However, these scales also have an important limitation: They generally provide only a single, global index of level of dependency (although in this context it must be noted that some projective oral dependency scales can also yield a separate index of preoccupation with food, eating, and other "oral" activities) (see Bornstein & Greenberg, 1991; Shilkret & Masling, 1981).

Masling et al.'s (1967) ROD scale is far and away the most widely used projective dependency measure. A description of the administration and scoring of this scale illustrates the kinds of procedures typically employed by researchers who utilize projective measures of dependency. Although the ROD can be administered individually or in groups, the most common form of the ROD is the group administration (Masling, 1986). In the group administration of the ROD, subjects are shown slides of the 10 Rorschach inkblots, in order, with each inkblot exposed for several minutes. Subjects are asked to write down two or three things that they see in each inkblot, with two responses to each inkblot requested for Cards IV, V, VI, VII, and IX, and three responses to each inkblot requested for the other five cards. Subjects' written descriptions are then scored for oral dependent content using a lexical system. Two categories of responses are used in ROD scoring: (1) dependent imagery (e.g., figures exhibiting overt dependent behavior, situations involving passivity and helplessness, nurturing and caretaking figures) and (2) oral imagery (i.e., food- and mouth-related percepts).

A detailed description of the categories used in ROD scoring is presented in Table 2.2. As Table 2.2 shows, categories 6, 9, 10, 11, 13, 14, and 15 represent "dependency-related" percepts, while categories 1, 2, 3, 4, 5, 7, 8, and 12 represent "oral" percepts. Percepts from category 16 can fall into either area, depending on the imagery contained in the percept. A discussion of the derivation, construction, and validation of this scale is provided by Masling (1986).

Subjects receive one point for each dependent or "oral" response on the ROD. Thus, ROD scores potentially range from 0 to 25, with higher scores indicating higher levels of oral dependency. In reality, ROD scores typically

**TABLE 2.2. Categories of Oral Dependent Responses on the ROD Scale**

| Category | Sample responses |
| --- | --- |
| 1. Foods and drinks | Milk, whiskey, boiled lobster |
| 2. Food sources | Restaurant, saloon, breast |
| 3. Food objects | Kettle, silverware, drinking glass |
| 4. Food providers | Waiter, cook, bartender |
| 5. Passive food receivers | Bird in nest, fat/thin man |
| 6. Begging and praying | Dogs begging, person saying prayers |
| 7. Food organs | Mouth, stomach, lips, teeth |
| 8. Oral instruments | Lipstick, cigarette, tuba |
| 9. Nurturers | Jesus, mother, father, doctor, God |
| 10. Gifts and gift givers | Christmas tree, cornucopia |
| 11. Good luck objects | Wishbone, four-leaf clover |
| 12. Oral activity | Eating, talking, singing, kissing |
| 13. Passivity and helplessness | Looking confused, lost |
| 14. Pregnancy and reproductive organs | Placenta, womb, ovaries, embryo |
| 15. "Baby talk" responses | Patty-cake, bunny rabbit, pussy cat |
| 16. Negations of oral dependent percepts | No mouth, woman with no breasts |

*Note.* In category 1, animals are scored only if they are invariably associated with eating (i.e., do not score "duck" or "turkey" unless food-descriptive phrases are used, such as "roast duck" or "turkey leg"). In category 3, "pot" and "cauldron" are scored only if the act of cooking is implied. In category 13, "baby" is only scored if there is some suggestion of passivity or frailness. In category 14, "pelvis," "penis," "vagina," and "sex organs" are not scored. Adapted from Bornstein and Masling (1985, Table 1). © 1985 by Lawrence Erlbaum Associates. Adapted by permission of the publisher.

range from 0 to 8. On rare occasions, a subject will report up to 10 or 11 oral dependent responses. Thus, the percentage of oral dependent responses typically produced on the ROD ranges from 0% to about 32%. In experiments that use the group-administered ROD to select subjects for study, nondependent subjects are operationally defined as those who produce two or fewer oral dependent responses (i.e., 8% or less), while dependent subjects are those who produce four or more oral dependent responses (i.e., 16% or more). Subjects who produce three oral dependent responses are dropped from the study. This subject selection procedure yields approximately equal numbers of dependent and nondependent subjects and has the additional advantage of identifying relatively "pure" dependent and non-dependent groups: The lowest scoring "dependent" subject gives twice as many oral dependent Rorschach responses as does the highest scoring "nondependent" subject.[1]

Because a lexical scoring system is used, interrater reliability in ROD scoring is very good, with independent raters almost invariably agreeing on the scoring of upwards of 90% of subjects' written responses (Bornstein &

Masling, 1985; Bornstein & Greenberg, 1991; Masling et al., 1967; Shil-kret & Masling, 1981). Not surprisingly, Pearson correlation coefficients between the ROD scores of two independent raters are generally higher than .90 (see, e.g., O'Neill & Bornstein, 1990, 1991).

## INTERVIEW AND RATING MEASURES

In a number of studies, dependency has been assessed via structured interview, behavioral observation, and peer, parent, teacher, or clinician ratings (e.g., Alnaes & Torgerson, 1988a, 1988b, 1990; Becker et al., 1962; Beller, 1955, 1957, 1959; Beswick & Cox, 1958; Crandall, Preston, & Rabson, 1960; Emmerich, 1964, 1966; Fitzgerald, 1958; Flanders, Anderson, & Amidon, 1961; Geshuri, 1975; Golightly, Nelson, & Johnson, 1970; Hart-up & Keller, 1960; Hedayat & Kelly, 1991; Kagan & Freeman, 1963; Kagan & Moss, 1960, 1962; Mann, 1959; Moskowitz, 1982; Nace, Davis & Gaspari, 1991; Sears, 1963; Sears et al., 1953; Sears & Wise, 1950; Shafar, 1976; Smith & Bain, 1978; Turner, 1991; Vaillant, 1974, 1978, 1980; Wiggins & Winder, 1961; Young & Smith, 1977; Zuckerman et al., 1961). These interview and rating techniques have certain advantages over other assessment methods, but they also present special problems for researchers. Interview and behavioral measures of dependency are considered separately.

### Interview Measures

Interview measures of dependency can be divided into two general categories. First, some researchers have used structured interviews designed to obtain information regarding an individual's dependency-related beliefs and behaviors. In most cases, such interviews are conducted with parents, who are asked to provide information regarding their child's dependent attitudes and behaviors (e.g., Kagan & Moss, 1960, 1962; Sears et al., 1953, 1957). However, in some studies subjects are interviewed directly (e.g., Kagan & Freeman, 1963; Vaillant, 1974, 1978, 1980), and in a few instances interviews are conducted with peers to obtain dependency-related information about a subject (e.g., Wiggins & Winder, 1961; Zuckerman et al., 1961).

The advantages of assessing dependency in children via parent interviews are obvious: Children—especially younger children—may not be able or willing to provide accurate self-reports of dependent behaviors. Moreover, parent interviews allow researchers to assess a wide variety of dependency-related behaviors in child subjects (e.g., help seeking, approval seeking), so that relationships among different aspects of dependent behavior can be examined. These interviews also permit researchers to assess developmental changes in children's dependent behaviors. Typically, this is accomplished in one of two ways. First, the parent may be asked to provide retrospective information regarding the child's behavior at different ages. Alternatively, repeated interviews with the parent may be conducted at different points in time, allowing longitudinal data to be collected directly.

Of course, interview rating techniques involve certain methodological problems and limitations. Most obviously, these measures are cumbersome, time-consuming, and relatively difficult to administer. Extensive training is often required to prepare the interviewers and raters who will be administering and scoring these measures. In this respect, interview measures of dependency are somewhat inefficient (not to mention expensive). However, a more serious methodological problem has to do with the validity of these measures. Parent-derived ratings of children's dependency may be distorted by selective memories for certain types of behavior, or by unintentional, unconscious revision and reconstruction of memories of parent–child interactions. Self-report and self-presentation biases may further distort parents' descriptions of their children's behavior. Similar self-presentation biases may also affect subjects' interview-based self-reports. Although the same kinds of problems potentially affect peer- or teacher-derived dependency ratings, self-presentation confounds will most likely affect teacher and peer ratings to a lesser extent than they influence parent ratings and subjects' self-reports.

The other area in which interviews are often used to assess dependency is in studies wherein DPD symptoms and diagnoses are assessed. In these investigations, structured clinical interviews based on DSM-III (APA, 1980) or DSM-III-R (APA, 1987) criteria are used to assess dependency (see Reich [1987a] for a detailed review of several widely used structured clinical interviews designed to obtain information regarding Axis II personality disorder symptoms). Typically, DPD patients are then compared to matched control patients (e.g., patients manifesting other Axis II diagnoses) on some criterion measure. Not surprisingly, the majority of these investigations are designed to examine the antecedents, correlates, and consequences of DPD diagnoses (e.g., Alnaes & Torgerson, 1988a, 1988b; Drake, Adler, & Vaillant, 1988; Reich, 1987b, 1987c). However, some studies in this area simply use DPD diagnoses or DPD symptom levels as a tool to select dependent subjects for study (e.g., Craig, 1988; Hayward & King, 1990; Poldrugo & Forti, 1988). Because interview raters in these investigations are generally blind to other information regarding the patients, and presumably have no motivation to present particular subjects in a positive (or negative) light, the possibility of self-report biases and other methodological confounds contaminating these ratings is minimized.

## Behavioral Measures

As might be expected, the majority of studies that employ behavioral measures of dependency have taken place either in the home or in school settings. These investigations almost invariably involve preschool, nursery school, or elementary school children (see, e.g., Beller, 1955, 1957, 1959; Beswick & Cox, 1958; Crandall et al., 1960; Kagan & Freeman, 1963; Kagan & Moss, 1960, 1962; Mann, 1959; Moskowitz, 1982; Sears, 1963; Smith & Bain, 1978; Turner, 1991; Watson, 1957; Young & Smith, 1977). Although the observers used in these studies to rate children's behavior usually are blind to the children's scores on relevant outcome measures (thus ensuring that behavioral observations are not contaminated by this information), there are two problems with the behavioral measures used to assess dependency in child subjects.

The first problem is methodological. Because the same observers assign ratings to each subject on a variety of dependency-related dimensions (e.g., help seeking, reassurance seeking), the observers are not blind to scores on different rating dimensions. Thus, it is possible that scores on a particular dependency-related subscale influence the ratings assigned on other subscales, creating a kind of "halo effect." Clearly, this would bias the dependency scores obtained when observational measures are used and would tend to inflate the intersubscale correlations that are obtained with these measures.

The second problem that characterizes behavioral measures of dependency has to do with the content of the behavioral dimensions that are included in these scales. Many observational measures of dependency assess proximity-seeking (i.e., attachment) behaviors as well as help- and reassurance-seeking (i.e., dependent) behaviors. Beller's (1955) behavioral rating system illustrates this confound. Beller's system includes teacher ratings of children's behavior in five areas: (1) help seeking; (2) contact seeking; (3) proximity seeking; (4) attention seeking; and (5) praise/reassurance/approval seeking. Although dimensions 1, 4, and 5 are clearly tapping dependency-related behaviors, dimensions 2 and 3 may be measuring something that is closer to attachment than to dependency (see Ainsworth, 1972; Livesley et al., 1990).

Similar confounds characterize Sears's (1963) behavioral rating system, wherein observers rate four categories of children's classroom behavior: (1) negative attention seeking; (2) positive attention seeking; (3) touching or holding; and (4) "being near" (i.e., proximity seeking). Only one of these dimensions (i.e., dimension 2) clearly taps dependency-related behaviors. In Sears's system, dimensions 3 and 4 appear to assess attachment-related behaviors, whereas dimension 1 assesses something that is neither dependency nor attachment. In fact, the behaviors that comprise dimension 1 of Sears's rating system (i.e., "disruption, aggressive activity with minimal provocation, defiance or oppositional behavior" [Sears, 1963, p. 32]) are closer to immature aggressiveness or hyperactivity than they are to dependency.

Insofar as behavioral rating systems such as those described by Bellers (1955), Sears (1963), and others confound dependency and attachment behaviors, it is difficult to tell the degree to which findings from these studies reflect differences in attachment style or differences in level of dependency. Fortunately, some recent behavioral rating systems (e.g., Geshuri, 1975) have corrected this problem, although others (e.g., Smith & Bain, 1978) continue to be compromised by dependency–attachment confounds. Needless to say, findings obtained using such measures must be interpreted cautiously.

## PSYCHOMETRIC ISSUES

Table 2.3 presents a brief description of the strengths and limitations of objective, projective, interview, and self-report measures of dependency. As Table 2.3 shows, each type of measure has certain advantages and certain disadvantages. In my view, projective measures have proved most useful in advancing our knowledge regarding the etiology, dynamics, and correlates of dependency, in part because the low face validity of these measures circumvents a number of self-report problems that can compromise studies of the dependent personality. Objective measures and interview measures of dependency have also yielded numerous important findings. Behavioral measures of dependency have been plagued by more methodological problems than have other types of measures, and have probably contributed less to this area of research than have other types of measures.

A detailed discussion of evidence regarding the psychometric properties of each dependency scale cited in this book is beyond the scope of this chapter. The articles listed in Table 2.1 discuss in detail findings regarding the psychometrics of the most widely used dependency scales, and the interested reader may want to examine these articles directly. However, the findings described in these papers can be summarized in general terms. For the most part, researchers have provided good evidence regarding the concurrent validity, convergent validity, discriminant validity, test–retest reliability, and (where appropriate) interrater reliability of their dependency measures. Researchers have been less attentive to issues regarding the predictive validity of their dependency scales. It is not the case that evidence regarding the predictive validity of these measures is weak. The problem is that there is little evidence at all regarding the predictive validity of these scales because researchers have almost invariably opted to collect depen-

**TABLE 2.3. Comparison of Different Types of Dependency Measures**

| Type of scale | Advantages | Disadvantages |
|---|---|---|
| Objective | 1. Easy to administer and score<br>2. Can yield subscores for different dimensions of dependency | 1. High face validity; easily "fakeable"<br>2. Taps "surface" only |
| Projective | 1. Low face validity; immune from self-report biases<br>2. Some projective tests provide alternate forms or subsets of stimuli, allowing for test–retest analysis<br>3. Taps latent/convert/unconscious traits | 1. Difficult to administer<br>2. Interrater reliablity can be a problem on some projective tests<br>3. Usually cannot provide information regarding dimensions of dependency |
| Interview | 1. Tester can probe or follow up on key areas<br>2. Can provide information in a wide variety of areas<br>3. Tester can assess verbal and nonverbal information during interview<br>4. Can yield life-history and time-sampling data | 1. Difficult to administer and score<br>2. Interrater reliability can be a problem<br>3. Self-report and self-presentation biases can be a problem |
| Rating/behavioral observation | 1. Yields measure of actual dependent behavior in a naturalistic setting<br>2. Provides information regarding a wide range of behavior, including interpersonal interaction *in vivo* | 1. Rater/observer bias can be a problem (e.g., halo effect can bias ratings)<br>2. Behavioral observation can be difficult to perform<br>3. Limited to certain settings, and to ratings of overt behavior |

dency-related information at the time that a scale was administered, rather than collecting outcome data at some later date.

In the following sections, I briefly discuss two issues related to the validity of various dependency measures. First, I review research examining the interrelationships among scores on different dependency scales. Second, I discuss the degree to which different dependency scales have produced consistent results in empirical studies of the dependent personality.

# Interrelationships of Scores on
## Different Dependency Scales

Relatively few studies have examined directly the concordance of scores on different dependency scales. Nonetheless, the results of studies conducted to date allow three general (albeit tentative) conclusions to be drawn regarding the interrelationships of scores on various dependency measures. First, as would be expected given the deleterious effects of method variance on interscale correlations, the correlations between measures within a particular category (e.g., objective, projective) are generally higher than are the correlations between measures that come from different categories. Typically, Pearson correlation coefficients between dependency scores that come from tests within a particular category are in the range of $r = .60-.80$ (see, e.g., Blaney & Kutcher, 1991; Blatt, Quinlan, Chevron, McDonald, & Zuroff, 1982; Masling et al., 1967; Sears et al., 1953; Wiggins & Winder, 1961), although some studies report slightly smaller correlation coefficients (e.g., Fitzgerald, 1958; Zuckerman et al., 1961).

Second, the correlations between dependency scores from objective tests and behavioral measures are somewhat higher than are other cross-category intertest correlations. It is not clear why this is so, but one possible explanation for these relatively high correlations has to do with the processes by which subjects generate responses to self-report measures of dependency. If subjects' responses to dependency-related questionnaire items are based in part on memories of dependent behaviors exhibited in social settings, then the relatively high correlations between self-report and behavioral measures of dependency may simply reflect the fact that both subject and observer are responding to the same kinds of information in generating ratings. Of course, this explanation requires empirical testing. At any rate, although these objective test–behavioral rating correlations vary considerably, they are typically in the $r = .40-.50$ range (see, e.g., Fu, Hinkle & Hanna, 1986; Golightly et al., 1970; Hedayat & Kelly, 1991).

Finally, correlations between dependency scores from projective tests and objective tests are somewhat lower than are the correlations typically obtained in other cross-category comparisons. This is probably due to differences in the face validity of objective and projective dependency scales. As my earlier discussion of the face validity of different dependency measures suggested (see also Table 2.3), it is likely that self-report and self-presentation biases affect subjects' responses to objective measures to a greater degree than they affect subjects' responses to projective measures, diminishing the correlation between scores obtained on dependency scales that come from these two categories. Nonetheless, correlations between scores on objective and projective dependency scales are generally statistically significant and in the predicted direction (see Bornstein, Poynton, & Masling, 1985; Masling et al., 1967; Sinha, 1968). Although there is considerable variability in the correlation coefficients obtained in these investigations, they typically fall into the $r = .30-.40$ range. However, a few studies have reported somewhat lower correlations between subjects' scores on objective and projective dependency scales (e.g., Bornstein et al., 1985), and some studies have reported somewhat higher correlations between objective and projective dependency scores (e.g., Sinha, 1968).

## Converging Results Obtained with Different Dependency Scales

Studies that assess directly the concordance of scores on different dependency scales support the convergent validity of these measures. The results of empirical studies of the dependent personality offer additional evidence that different types of dependency measures are in fact assessing a common personality dimension. As the ensuing review of the empirical literature on dependency demonstrates, investigations using different dependency measures have yielded consistent findings. Specifically, in studies of parenting style, suggestibility, interpersonal compliance, help seeking, interpersonal sensitivity, affiliative behavior, verbal conditioning, performance anxiety, sociometric status, jealousy, depression, phobias, alcoholism, smoking, eating disorders, physical disorders, treatment delay, and treatment duration, different types of dependency measures (e.g., objective vs. projective, oral dependency scales vs measures of interpersonal dependency) have yielded highly similar results. Clearly, additional work remains to be done to examine more completely the similarities and differences among different dependency measures. However, the finding that different types of dependency measures produce similar results is inconsistent with earlier suggestions that "overt" (i.e., objective) and "covert" (projective) measures of dependency assess different dimensions of personality (Diener, 1967; Zuckerman et al., 1961).

## NOTE

1. A slightly different scoring system must be used when ROD scores are derived from individually administered Rorschach tests. In this situation, different subjects produce different numbers of responses to the inkblots. To control for the effects of response productivity on ROD scores, the percentage of oral dependent responses (i.e., the number of oral dependent responses divided by the total number of responses [R]) is calculated when ROD scores are derived from individually administered Rorschach protocols.

# The Development
# of Dependency

A great deal of effort has gone into research examining various factors that are hypothesized to underly the epigenesis of dependency in infancy and early childhood. Studies conducted to date do not suggest that dependency has a strong genetic linkage (see Buss, 1983; Dworkin, Burke, Maher, & Gottesman, 1976; Freedman, 1971; Maccoby & Masters, 1970). Consequently, the vast majority of studies examining the etiology and development of dependency have focused on environmental variables. In this chapter, I discuss research examining (1) the epigenesis of dependency in infancy and early childhood, (2) the stability of dependent personality traits from childhood through adulthood, (3) sex differences in dependency, and (4) the relationship of dependency to sex-role orientation.

## THE EPIGENESIS OF DEPENDENCY

Studies of the epigenesis of dependency can be divided into two areas. First, a number of researchers have tested the psychoanalytic hypothesis that childhood, adolescent, and adult dependency can be traced to feeding and weaning experiences during infancy. Second, a number of researchers have taken a somewhat broader view, examining the relationship between various aspects of the parent–child relationship and later dependency. Research in these two areas will be considered separately.[1]

### Feeding/Weaning Variables as Predictors
### of Later Dependency

During the 1940s, 1950s, and 1960s, numerous researchers investigated the relationship of infantile feeding and weaning experiences to later dependency. The general approach used in these studies involved obtaining retrospective reports of feeding and weaning behaviors from the mother and assessing the relationship of various feeding and weaning variables (i.e., duration of breastfeeding, rigidity of feeding schedule, breast- vs. bottle feeding, severity of weaning) to some measure of childhood or adult dependency (see Goldman-Eisler, 1948, 1950, 1951; Heinstein, 1963; Sears, 1963; Sears et al., 1953, 1965; Sears, Maccoby, & Levin, 1957; Sears & Wise, 1950; Stendler, 1954; Thurston & Mussen, 1951). Although there was some variation in the specific hypotheses tested in different investigations, there was enough overlap among these hypotheses that they can be summarized in general terms. Researchers investigating the feeding/weaning–dependency relationship hypothesized that exaggerated dependency needs in childhood or adulthood would result from (1) either a very long (i.e., "overgratifying") or very brief (i.e., "frustrating") nursing period; (2) a rigid (as opposed to flexible) feeding schedule; (3) bottle feeding rather than breastfeeding; and (4) "severe" (i.e., abrupt) weaning.

One of the most extensive early studies in this area was conducted by Sears et al. (1953), who examined the relationship of several indices of infantile feeding and weaning practices (e.g., mothers' reports of rigidity of feeding schedule and severity of weaning) to various measures of childhood dependency (e.g., teachers' ratings, observers' ratings of dependent behavior exhibited in the classroom) in a mixed-sex sample of 40 nursery school children. One important strength of this study was the use of multiple measures of dependent behavior, which allowed the investigators to examine interrelationships among different outcome measures. In addition, Sears et al. were careful to establish the construct validity of the dependency measures used in this investigation, and provided detailed information regarding the convergent and discriminant validity of the different indices of dependent behavior.

Sears et al. (1953) found that the relationship between rigidity of infantile feeding schedule and later dependency was different in boys and girls. Specifically, although the correlation between rigidity of feeding and teacher-rated dependency was marginally significant for girls ($r = .31$), no comparable relationship was found for boys ($r = .07$). Somewhat stronger results were found for the relationship of severity of weaning to teacher-rated dependency, where correlations were .47 for girls and .39 for boys. No significant relationships were found between feeding or weaning variables and classroom-observed dependency.

Although Sears et al.'s (1953) initial findings regarding the dependency–severity of weaning relationship seemed promising, they were never replicated. In fact, when Sears et al. (1957) conducted a large-scale follow-up of their earlier study, this time collecting data from a sample of 379 kindergarten children, they found no consistent relationship between various feeding and weaning variables and multiple measures of dependency taken around age 4. Level of dependency was unrelated to severity of weaning in Sears et al.'s (1957) sample. Furthermore, Sears et al.'s (1957) findings regarding the relationship of dependency to rigidity of feeding schedule were precisely the opposite of what they had found in their earlier study: There was a slight (but statistically significant) inverse relationship between rigidity of feeding schedule and ratings of dependency for boys ($r = -.17$), with rigid feeding schedules associated with *lower* levels of dependency. No comparable relationship was found for girls.

The results of other studies in this area were not much more encouraging. For example, Thurston and Mussen (1951) found no relationship whatsoever between mothers' retrospective reports of several feeding and weaning variables and their adolescent children's level of dependency assessed via the TAT. Thurston and Mussen examined the relationship between three feeding/weaning variables (i.e., age of weaning, rigidity of feeding schedule, breast- vs bottle feeding) and 30 TAT indices of dependency. This yielded 90 separate dependency–feeding/weaning comparisons. Four of the 90 comparisons were significant at $p < .05$, which is almost exactly what would have been expected on the basis of chance alone. Consistent with Thurston and Mussen's results, Stendler (1954) found no relationship between age of weaning or difficulty in weaning and teachers' ratings of level of dependency at age 5. Sears (1963) and Sears et al. (1965) also found no strong or consistent relationships between various infantile feeding and weaning variables and observational measures of childhood dependency.

Finally, Heinstein's (1963) large-scale longitudinal study of the relationship of early feeding experiences to later dependency also failed to produce consistent results. Heinstein examined the relationship of two feeding variables (i.e., breast- vs. bottle feeding and length of the nursing period) to several indices of later dependency (i.e., preschool and late childhood ratings of dependency, TAT dependency scores, Rorschach oral dependency scores) in a mixed-sex sample of 252 children. Separate analyses were conducted for boys and girls. Of the 16 comparisons between predictor and criterion variables in Heinstein's study, one produced results significant at $p < .05$: Breast-fed boys had significantly higher TAT dependency scores in late childhood (i.e., between ages 9 and 11) than did bottle-fed boys.

Examination of the nonsignificant trends obtained in Heinstein's (1963) investigation is informative because it illustrates the confusing and inconsistent patterns of relationships between feeding and weaning variables and later dependency that are obtained even in carefully designed longitudinal studies of this issue. Table 3.1 summarizes Heinstein's findings, noting the trends between (1) method of feeding (i.e., breast vs. bottle) and later dependency and (2) length of nursing period (i.e., age of weaning) and later dependency. As this table shows, the results obtained for boys and girls are inconsistent with respect to method of feeding. For boys, it appears that breastfeeding may be associated with higher levels of dependency, while for girls, the opposite is true. Furthermore, while dependency in boys appears to be predicted by a long period of nursing, for girls the relationship between length of nursing and later dependency is more complex and may change over time. In fact, Heinstein's results suggest that a long period of nursing is associated with elevated dependency in girls during childhood, while a short period of nursing is associated with elevated dependency in girls during adolescence.

Although studies in this area have produced inconclusive results, one important methodological limitation of these investigations warrants mention because it might well account for some or all of the nonsignificant findings reported in studies of infantile feeding and later dependency. As noted earlier, all studies in this area relied on mothers' retrospective reports of feeding and weaning practices. While some of the feeding/weaning data collected from mothers consisted of objective information (e.g., reports of

**TABLE 3.1. Summary of Heinstein's Findings Regarding the Relationship of Infantile Feeding and Weaning Variables to Later Dependency**

| Measure of dependency | Variable associated with increased dependency | |
|---|---|---|
| | Boys | Girls |
| Breast versus bottle feeding | | |
| Preschool dependency rating | Bottle | Bottle |
| Late childhood dependency rating | Breast | Bottle |
| Rorschach orality score | Breast | Bottle |
| TAT dependency score | Breast | Bottle |
| Length of nursing | | |
| Preschool dependency rating | Long | Long |
| Late childhood dependency rating | Long | Long |
| Rorschach orality score | Long | Short |
| TAT dependency score | Long | Short |

*Note.* The relationship between method of feeding and TAT dependency score in boys was significant at $p = .05$; all other relationships described in this table are nonsignificant trends. Preschool dependency ratings were obtained when the child subjects were between 21 and 42 months old. Late childhood dependency ratings were obtained when the child subjects were between 9 and 11 years old. Rorschach and TAT protocols were collected when the subjects were between 21 and 42 months old. Late childhood dependency ratings were obtained when the child subjects were between 9 and 11 years old. Rorschach and TAT protocols were collected when the subjects were 18 years old. Adapted from Heinstein (1963, Tables 4 and 5). © 1963 by the Society for Research in Child Development. Adapted by permission of the publisher.

breast- vs. bottle feeding, information regarding length of the nursing period), other data involved more subjective judgments on the part of mothers (e.g., judgments of rigidity of feeding schedule). The problem is this: It is not clear that mothers can provide accurate self-reports with respect to these "soft" variables, for several reasons.

First, "rigidity of feeding" is difficult to define operationally; idiosyncratic interpretations of this variable—on the part of both examiner and subject—could have diminished the predictive validity of these ratings. Second, it is likely that the mother's ongoing interactions with her child influenced her memories of past mother–child interactions, so that memories of subjective experiences such as rigidity of feeding schedule might not have been accurate. Third, even if mothers' memories for such information as rigidity of feeding schedule were accurate, self-presentation bias, need for approval, and numerous other factors potentially compromise the accuracy of these reports.

The accuracy of mothers' retrospective reports of rigidity of feeding schedule turns out to be a critical issue. As the ensuing review of the literature on parent–child interactions as predictors of later dependency will show, rigidity of feeding schedule might well be the feeding/weaning variable with the best potential to predict later dependency.

## The Parent–Child Relationship as a Predictor of Later Dependency

Studies assessing the influence of the overall infant–caretaker relationship on later dependency and studies examining differences in parenting style of parents of dependent and nondependent children have produced consistent findings[2] (see Bandura & Walters, 1959; Baumrind, 1967, 1971; Baumrind & Black, 1967; Becker et al., 1962; Berg & McGuire, 1974; Bhogle, 1983; Bird, Martin, & Schuham, 1983; Crandall et al., 1960; Finney, 1961; Gordon & Tegtemeyer, 1983; Hatfield, Ferguson, Rau, & Alpert, 1967; Head, Baker, & Williamson, 1991; Heathers, 1953; Levy, 1943; McCord, McCord, & Thurber, 1962; Murphy, 1962; Ojha & Singh, 1988; Parker, 1979a, 1979b; Parker & Lipscombe, 1980; Roe & Siegelman, 1963; Sears, 1963; Sears et al., 1957, 1965; Siegelman, 1966; Smith, 1958; Sroufe et al., 1983; Stendler, 1954; Watson, 1934, 1957; Whiffen & Sasseville, 1991; Wickstrom & Fleck, 1983; Winder & Rau, 1962). Furthermore, investigations in this area have used a wide variety of measures and methodologies (e.g., retrospective reports of parenting practices, direct observations of parent–child interactions, assessments of parental perceptions in adolescent subjects). Because these studies produced consistent results despite using different measures and procedures, strong conclusions can be drawn from the results of these investigations.

In one of the most extensive and well-designed studies in this area, Finney (1961) interviewed the mothers of 31 boys enrolled in a child guidance clinic, obtaining information regarding a variety of dimensions related to the infant–mother relationship (e.g., maternal protectiveness, rigidity of discipline, expression of affection). Clinicians' ratings of the mothers on these same dimensions were also obtained. Clinicians' and teachers' ratings were used to assess level of dependency in the child subjects. The mothers of dependent boys differed from the mothers of nondependent boys in that they were significantly more protective of their child. Specifically, significant correlations were obtained between maternal protectiveness ratings and the child's dependency score ($r = .37$), and between ratings of a mother's tendency to reinforce dependent behavior and her child's dependency score ($r = .40$). Similar results were obtained by Baumrind (1967, 1971), Berg and McGuire (1974), Crandall et al. (1960), Gordon and Tegtemeyer (1983), Hatfield et al. (1967), Head et al. (1991), Heathers (1953), Murphy (1962), Sears et al. (1957), Smith (1958), and Stendler (1954). These results echo Levy's (1943) earlier finding that maternal overprotectiveness predicted the later expression of dependency in adolescent boys.

Studies of parenting style that used retrospective reports obtained from parents and their (adult) children produced results generally consistent with those of Levy (1943), Finney (1961), and others. For example, Ojha and Singh (1988) found that parental overprotectiveness (assessed via Ojha's [1972] Parental Behavior Inventory) was associated with increased dependency (assessed via Sinha's [1968] DP scale) in college student subjects. Parker and Lipscombe (1980) similarly found that reports of parental overprotectiveness (assessed via Parker, Tupling, & Brown's [1979] Parental Bonding Instrument) were associated with increased dependency (assessed via the DEQ dependency scale [Blatt et al., 1976]) in a mixed-sex sample of adult medical patients. Similar results were also obtained by Bird et al. (1983) and Richman and Flaherty (1987), who examined the parental overprotectiveness–dependency relationship in samples of psychiatric outpatients and medical students.

While a number of studies found parental overprotectiveness to be associated with increased dependency in children, adolescents, and adults, several studies also found parental authoritarianism to predict later dependency. For example, Vaillant (1980) found that memories of the parents as harsh and demanding during childhood were associated with elevated levels of dependency in a sample of 184 male undergraduates who were first studied around age 20 and then reassessed at age 50. Similarly, McCranie and Bass (1984) found that ratings of parental "strict control" (assessed via Kelly & Worrell's [1976] Parental Behavior Form) were positively correlated with DEQ dependency scores in a sample of 86 female undergraduates. Consistent with these results, Baumrind (1967, 1971), Bhogle (1983), McCord et al. (1962), McPartland and Epstein (1975), Roe and Siegelman (1963), Watson (1934, 1957), Whiffen and Sasseville (1991), and Winder and Rau (1962) found that parental authoritarianism and authoritarian parenting styles were associated with increased dependency during early, middle, and late childhood.[3]

Wickstrom and Fleck (1983) took a slightly different approach to this issue, assessing the parenting styles of mothers and fathers separately. They found different patterns of parental relationships in dependent males and females. Dependent male college students in Wickstrom and Fleck's sample reported significantly lower levels of maternal acceptance and significantly higher levels of maternal control than did nondependent male subjects. In contrast, dependent females reported higher levels of paternal acceptance than did nondependent females. However, no differences in the maternal relationship were found for dependent versus nondependent females.

Wickstrom and Fleck's (1983) results for male subjects parallel those of Bornstein, Galley, and Leone (1986), who found that dependent male college students (selected according to scores on Masling et al.'s [1967] ROD scale) described the mother—but not the father—as significantly less nurturant, benevolent, warm, and constructively involved than did nondependent males. In addition, dependent males in Bornstein et al.'s sample described the mother as significantly more punitive than did nondependent males. Consistent with the findings of Wickstrom and Fleck, there was no relationship between level of dependency and perceptions of the father in Bornstein et al.'s sample of male college students. Thus, the results of Wickstrom and Fleck's and Bornstein et al.'s studies suggest that the child's relationship with the opposite-sex parent may be more influential than the child's relationship with the same-sex parent in determining later dependency.

Results from studies of parent–child interactions, investigations of parenting style, and studies of parental perceptions in adult subjects suggest that parental overprotectiveness and authoritarianism play a significant role in determining level of dependency. Highly consistent results in this area were obtained in independent samples of American (Kagan & Moss, 1960; McCranie & Bass, 1984), Indian (Bhogle, 1983; Ojha & Singh, 1988), and British subjects (Berg & McGuire, 1974; Parker & Lipscombe, 1980), despite the fact that these studies employed different measures and procedures. The cross-cultural and cross-methodological consistency of results regarding the dependency–parenting style relationship attests to the robustness and generalizability of these findings.[4]

Nonetheless, findings regarding the relationship of parenting style to the development of dependency in children raise two important (and related) questions. First, do overprotective parents tend to use authoritarian parenting practices or are parental overprotectiveness and authoritarianism orthogonal (i.e., independent, unrelated) traits? Second, what is the link between parental overprotectiveness and authoritarianism and the development of dependent personality traits in children?

Baumrind's (1967, 1971; Baumrind & Black, 1967) studies of the interrelationships among various dimensions of parenting style help to address the first question. Although Baumrind found some degree of overlap between parental overprotectiveness and authoritarianism (i.e., a slight positive correlation between parental overprotectiveness and authoritarianism ratings on certain behavioral dimensions), her results suggest that overall, parental overprotectiveness and authoritarianism are best conceptualized as orthogonal traits (see also Baumrind [1973] for a detailed discussion of these findings and their implications). Although there may be some tendency for overprotective parents to use authoritarian parenting practices, in any given sample of parents it is possible to identify individuals who are high in overprotectiveness and low in authoritarianism (or vice versa). Moreover, the "authoritative" parents in Baumrind's samples did not show particularly high levels of either of these characteristics. Thus, parents can be divided into four categories with respect to overprotectiveness and authoritarianism: (1) overprotective and authoritarian; (2) overprotective but not authoritarian; (3) authoritarian but not overprotective; and (4) not overprotective and not authoritarian.

The question remains: What is the link between parental overprotectiveness and authoritarianism and the development of dependent personality traits in children? Parental overprotectiveness and authoritarianism serve simultaneously to (1) reinforce dependent behaviors in children of both sexes and (2) prevent the child from developing independent, autonomous behaviors (since the parents do not permit the child to engage in the kinds of trial-and-error learning that are involved in developing a sense of independence and mastery during childhood) (see Bandura & Walters, 1959, 1963; Baumrind, 1973; Walters & Parke, 1964). Thus, when parental overprotectiveness *or* parental authoritarianism is characteristic of the family unit, this will tend to produce high levels of dependency in children (since both parenting styles foster and encourage dependent behavior). When *both* parental overprotectiveness and parental authoritarianism are present within the family unit, dependency in children is particularly likely to result.[5]

Extensive discussions of the relationship between reinforcement of dependent behavior in children and later dependency are provided by Bandura and Walters (1963) and Mischel (1970). In addition, the results of studies by Becker et al. (1961), Berg and McGuire (1974), Baumrind (1967, 1971), Baumrind and Black (1967), Cairns (1962), Crandall et al. (1960), Finney (1961), Fu et al. (1984), McCord et al. (1962), Sears (1963), Sears et al. (1965), and Sroufe et al. (1983) offer strong support for the hypothesis that reinforcement of dependent behavior in children produces high levels of dependency. In each of these investigations, parental reinforcement of dependent behavior (or punishment of independent behavior) during early childhood predicted level of dependency during later childhood and/or adolescence.

In a particularly well-designed longitudinal study of dependency and parenting style, Fu et al. (1986) assessed level of dependency and childrearing attitudes and behaviors in a sample of 150 grandmother–mother–child family "units" (in every case, the primary caretaker in these rural Appalachian families was the mother). Consistent with the findings of Cairns (1961) and others, Fu et al. found that reinforcement of dependent behavior in early childhood predicted level of dependency in late childhood, adolescence and adulthood. Three findings in particular are relevant in the present context. First, dependency-fostering behavior in the grandmothers predicted level of dependency in their adult daughters (i.e., the mothers in Fu et al.'s sample). Second, dependency-fostering behavior in the mothers predicted childhood and adolescent dependency in the daughters. Third, Fu et al. found that dependent caretakers were more likely than nondependent caretakers to reinforce dependent behaviors in their children, and to have overprotective, authoritarian childrearing attitudes. Despite the fact that Fu et al. only studied female caretakers and children in this study, their findings suggest that dependency may be "transmitted" across successive generations by overprotective, authoritarian parenting and by direct reinforcement of dependent behaviors in children.

Although results in this area indicate that parental authoritarianism and overprotectiveness predict the development of dependent behaviors in children, one important caveat regarding this conclusion must be kept in mind: While the links between overprotective, authoritarian parenting and later dependency are clearly supported by the results of relevant empirical studies, some investigations suggest that other parenting practices may also be associated with increased dependency in children. The relationship between these parenting practices and the development of dependency in children is less firmly established than is the relationship between overprotective, authoritarian parenting and later dependency. Nonetheless, several findings in this area are noteworthy. First, Baumrind and Black (1967) found that parental permissiveness was associated with high levels of dependency in preschool children. Second, Baumrind (1971) and Whiffen and Sasseville (1991) found that parental conformity predicted dependency in preschool children and college students. Finally, several researchers (e.g., Egeland & Sroufe, 1981; McCord et al., 1962; Smith, 1958; Wittenborn, 1956) found that parental neglect, rejection, and maltreatment produced high levels of dependency in children of various ages.

At first glance, these findings appear to contradict the results of studies which indicate that parental overprotectiveness and authoritarianism lead to the development of dependency in children. However, it is important to note that each of these behavior patterns (i.e., permissiveness, conformity, and abusiveness/neglect) is associated with reinforcement of passive, dependent behavior in children and with the discouragement of independent, autonomous functioning (see Maccoby, 1980; Maccoby & Masters, 1970). In this respect, these parental traits and behaviors would be expected to have similar effects on children's dependency levels as do parental overprotectiveness and authoritarianism. Clearly, the common link among various parenting practices that produce high levels of dependency in children is that these parenting practices indirectly encourage and reinforce dependent behavior in the child.

What, then, are we to make of the results of several investigations which suggest that forcing children to be highly independent at a very early age also produces increased dependency during middle and late childhood (see, e.g., Hatfield et al., 1967; Sears, 1963; Sears et al., 1965; Whiting & Child, 1953)? On the surface, these results seem to be in direct opposition to the oft-reported finding that parental overprotectiveness and reinforcement of dependent behavior produce high levels of dependency in children. However, scrutiny of these results indicates that they are in fact quite consistent with other findings in this area. When parents overemphasize independent achievement before the child is cognitively and emotionally prepared to deal with such demands, the child is placed under considerable pressure to perform behaviors that are beyond his or her capabilities. Not surprisingly, a child placed under such pressure cannot cope with parental demands and expectations, develops a view of him- or herself as inadequate and ineffectual, looks to others for guidance and support, and as a consequence, continues to display the kinds of passive, dependent behaviors that characterize earlier stages of development.

Parker (1960) provided an excellent summary of the processes by which premature demands for independence produce high levels of dependency in children. He argued:

> [W]hen the normal dependency needs of the immature child . . . are frustrated, and he is forced to assume tasks for which there is but little preparation in terms of his own self-confidence and ego strength, he tends to perpetuate his view of his parents as omnipotent and omniscient figures. Accordingly, he develops "magical" expectations of support and aid from them. This compensates for his own feelings of inadequacy. Essentially, the self-esteem, confidence and ego resources of the dependent person have been damaged and he is forced to endow others with the power that he feels he lacks. (p. 607)

Two decades earlier, Kardiner (1939) had developed a similar argument, explicitly linking cultural norms regarding early socialization practices with the inadvertent propagation of dependency needs in children, adolescents, and adults.

Thus, just as parental overprotectiveness and authoritarianism prevent the child from engaging in the kinds of trial-and-error learning that are critical for the development of a sense of autonomy and self-confidence, unrealistic independence and achievement expectations on the part of the parents can result in the child's continuing to display high levels of passive, dependent behavior during middle and late childhood. Not surprisingly, parents who impose unrealistic demands regarding independence and achievement on their children also tend to obtain high scores on indices of authoritarianism and authoritarian parenting practices (Baumrind, 1973). In effect, results regarding the influence of parental "overemphasis on autonomy and achievement" on children's dependency are simply another example of the ways in which parental authoritarianism may foster dependent behavior in children (see also Barry, Barry, & Lindemann [1965] and Birtchnell [1980] for findings regarding the relationship of premature demands for independence and later dependency in subjects who suffered early maternal bereavement).

One final caveat regarding the parenting style–dependency relationship warrants mention: Although overprotective, authoritarian parenting practices may encourage the development of dependent behaviors in children, it is also true that dependent behaviors exhibited by the child serve to encourage and reinforce overprotectiveness and authoritarianism in the parents. A number of studies have demonstrated that dependent behaviors exhibited by children elicit strong protective behaviors in both mothers and fathers (e.g., Hunt, Browning, & Nave, 1982; Marcus, 1975, 1976; Osofsky & O'Connell, 1972; cf. Parker, 1981). Other studies have demonstrated that dependent behaviors in children can result in increased parental demandingness (see Kaul et al., 1982). Thus, while the epigenesis of dependency may well lie in parental overprotectiveness and authoritarianism, the relationship between child dependency and parental behavior is synergistic and characterized by mutual influence and reciprocal reinforcement.

Clearly, additional longitudinal data are needed to clarify the causal relationship between parenting practices and childhood dependency. In this context, researchers may want to examine the possibility that infantile temperament variables (e.g., adaptability, responsiveness, soothability [see Rothbart, 1981; Thomas & Chess, 1977]) mediate the parenting style–dependency relationship. There has been relatively little research examining the possibility that infantile temperament variables predict later dependency, although it is clear that infants' (and children's) temperament-related behaviors affect parents' approaches to childrearing in important ways (Buss & Plomin, 1984).

There are at least two plausible routes whereby individual differences in infantile temperament could lead to high levels of childhood dependency. First, it may be that variations in infantile temperament lead to predictable patterns of parenting, which in turn affect children's dependency levels. This would represent an indirect temperament–dependency link wherein temperament-induced changes in parenting style affect the development of dependent personality traits in the child. Alternatively, it is possible that certain temperament variables (e.g., low adaptability, low soothability) gradually evolve into more complex dependent behaviors (e.g., help seeking, need for reassurance) as the child's behavioral repertoire increases. This latter framework would suggest that there is a direct link between infantile temperament and childhood dependency. Regardless of whether either of these developmental frameworks ultimately proves useful in conceptualizing the etiology and development of dependent personality traits in childhood, research assessing possible temperament–dependency links will allow researchers to reexamine the interesting possibility that dependent personality traits are to some degree determined by genetic factors: To the extent that dependency-related variations in temperament are attributable to inherited predispositions (see Buss & Plomin, 1984; Millon, 1981; Thomas & Chess, 1977), dependency itself might also be traceable in part to genetic factors.

## EVALUATING THE PSYCHOANALYTIC AND SOCIAL LEARNING MODELS WITH RESPECT TO THE ETIOLOGY OF DEPENDENCY

Although findings regarding the role of early socialization experiences in the etiology of dependency are consistent with the social learning model, it might be premature to interpret these findings as contradicting the classical psychoanalytic view of dependency as rooted in experiences that occur during the infantile, oral phase of development. While it is true that studies of dependency and infantile feeding and weaning behaviors have produced inconsistent, inconclusive findings, two methdological limitations of these studies prevent us from drawing strong conclusions from their results. The first important limitation of studies in this area was discussed earlier: The accuracy of mothers' retrospective reports of behaviors such as rigidity of feeding schedule is, to say the least, questionable.

Another important limitation of these studies involves researchers' failure to assess the possible influence of parental overprotectiveness and authoritarianism on feeding and weaning practices. As Maccoby (1980) noted, it is likely that the same qualities of the parent–child relationship that predict later dependency (i.e., overprotectiveness and authoritarianism) would also be manifest in the mother's early feeding and weaning behaviors.

In other words, authoritarian parenting (in general) should be associated with an authoritarian feeding and weaning style. Similarly, parental over-protectiveness should be associated with particular patterns of feeding and weaning behaviors. Unfortunately, the possibility that an overprotective or authoritarian parenting style influences infantile feeding and weaning practices has never been tested directly.

This brings us back to the first problem characterizing studies of the feeding/weaning–dependency relationship, because the feeding/weaning variable that seems most likely to be influenced by authoritarian parenting practices is rigidity of feeding schedule. It is reasonable to assume that authoritarian parents are less flexible in their feeding practices than are parents who are less authoritarian. However, until (1) the relationship of parental authoritarianism to rigidity of feeding schedule is assessed directly and (2) researchers examine directly the accuracy of mothers' retrospective reports of various feeding and weaning practices, it will be difficult to draw strong conclusions regarding the predictive validity of the psychoanalytic model with respect to the etiology of dependency.

## DEPENDENCY, GENDER, AND SEX ROLE

Psychologists and laypersons alike have long assumed that women are more dependent than men. In fact, this belief is so pervasive within the scientific and lay communities that it would be difficult to find someone who does not ascribe to this assumption (see Gilbert, 1987; Lerner, 1983). Of course, the question of whether there are gender differences in dependency is really an empirical one. Happily, a great deal of data are available that address this question directly. These data do not always support widely held cultural stereotypes regarding sex differences in dependency. In the following sections, I review research on sex differences in dependency, studies of the stability of dependency from childhood through adulthood, and studies of the relationship of dependency to sex-role orientation.

### Sex and Age Differences in Dependency

The likelihood that sex differences in dependency will be obtained in any given study is a function of the type of dependency measure used in that investigation. When self-report measures of dependency are used, the vast majority of studies examining gender differences in adult dependency have found significantly higher levels of dependency in women than in men (e.g., Banu & Puhan, 1983; Conley, 1980; Evans, 1984; Hedayat & Kelly, 1991; Lao, 1980; Ojha & Singh, 1985; Overholser, Kabakoff, & Norman, 1989; Selvey, 1973; Steele, 1978; Tripathi, 1982; Vats, 1986; Whiffen & Sasseville, 1991). Similar gender differences in dependency are found in school-age children when self-report measures are used (Chadha, 1983; Golightly et al., 1970; Ojha & Singh, 1972). Furthermore, comparable gender differences on self-report dependency measures are found in American (Chevron, Quinlan, & Blatt, 1978), British (Birtchnell & Kennard, 1983), German (Ederer, 1988), Japanese (Fujihara & Kurokawa, 1981), and Indian subjects (Singh & Ojha, 1987).

In contrast, when projective measures of dependency are employed, researchers typically find that men and women (and boys and girls) show similar levels of dependency (Bornstein, O'Neill, Galley, Leone, & Castrianno, 1988b; Fisher, 1970; Gordon & Tegtemeyer, 1983; Greenberg & Bornstein, 1989; Juni, Masling, & Brannon, 1979; Lansky, Crandall, Kagan, & Baker, 1961; Mills & Cunningham, 1988; Shilkret & Masling, 1981; Weiss, 1969; Weiss & Masling, 1970). These patterns are found in both normal (i.e., nonclinical) subjects (Bornstein, Leone, & Galley, 1988a) and psychiatric inpatients and outpatients (O'Neill & Bornstein, 1990). In short, women report higher levels of dependency than do men on self-report measures, but men and women obtain comparable dependency scores on projective measures.[6]

What accounts for the different patterns of results produced by self-report and projective dependency measures? The most likely explanation has to do with the face validity of the measures. As noted in Chapter 2, self-report measures of dependency ask the subject to respond to direct questions about dependent traits, feelings, and behaviors. Clearly, men will be less willing than women to acknowledge dependent traits and feelings, even if they are aware of them. However, projective measures of dependency (e.g., the ROD, TAT, or HIT) ask subjects for open-ended descriptions of ambiguous stimuli such as inkblots or drawings. These open-ended descriptions are then scored for dependent (or oral dependent) content, but of course the subjects are unaware of what content areas are of interest to the experimenter. Consequently, subjects will be unable to disguise or distort their projective test responses based on social desirability and self-presentation needs. Thus, despite the fact that subjects' scores on self-report and projective measures of dependency are generally positively intercorrelated (Bornstein et al., 1985; Fitzgerald, 1958; Sinha, 1968), self-report measures consistently yield substantially greater sex differences in dependency scores than do projective measures.

It is informative to contrast the findings obtained regarding gender differences in dependency in adults with the findings obtained in studies of children. Longitudinal studies of dependency in children typically find little or no difference in boys' and girls' dependency levels during early childhood (Maccoby & Jacklin, 1974; Maccoby & Masters, 1970; Mischel, 1970; Sears, 1963; Sears et al., 1957). However, gender differences in dependency increase with increasing age (Golightly et al., 1970; Kagan & Moss, 1960, 1962), and by the time children reach puberty, girls almost invariably show significantly higher dependency levels than do boys on self-report measures (Chadha, 1983; Moran & Carter, 1991; Yeger & Miezitis, 1985).

Kagan and Moss's (1960) classic longitudinal study of dependency illustrates the general pattern of results obtained in most investigations of this issue. Kagan and Moss utilized (1) in-home observations of infant-mother interactions to assess qualities of the infant–mother relationship and (2) interview, self-report, and observational measures to assess level of dependency during childhood and adulthood. They found that childhood dependency scores were significantly better predictors of dependency scores in adulthood for women than for men. The mean correlation between combined dependency scores at ages 6–10 and self-ratings of dependency on parents and romantic partners at ages 20–29 was .45 for women and .10 for men (see also Block [1971] for some related findings regarding this issue).

Golightly et al.'s (1970) results further suggest that gender differences in self-reported dependency begin to reveal themselves by middle to late childhood. Using a cross-sectional design, Golightly et al. assessed self-reported dependency in samples of fourth, fifth, and sixth graders using the Children's Dependency Scale (CDS). They found no sex differences in mean CDS scores in their 4th-grade sample, but found significant sex differences in CDS scores in the 5th and 6th graders. Furthermore, there was an overall trend toward increasing sex differences with increasing grade level in Golightly et al.'s sample: Boys' CDS scores showed a more rapid decrease with increasing age than did girls' CDS scores. Of course, longitudinal data would have provided more compelling evidence regarding developmental trends in self-reported dependency than do these cross-sectional data. Nonetheless, Golightly et al.'s results suggest that the gender differences in self-reported dependency typically observed in men and women are detectable by around age 9 or 10.

Golightly et al.'s (1970) findings raise an important question: What accounts for the increasing gender differences in self-reported dependency that are apparent by middle to late childhood? To address this issue, we must examine (1) the patterns of dependency scores that are obtained by subjects of different ages and (2) the specific behaviors that characterize dependency at different ages.

Several investigators have found that in general, children's scores on various dependency measures tend to decrease with increasing age (see, e.g., Boehm, 1947; Heathers, 1953; Stith & Connor, 1962; Wiggins & Winder, 1961). Although there has not yet been a definitive longitudinal study of developmental changes in boys' and girls' dependency levels, it appears that gender differences in dependency emerge by around age 9 or 10 primarily because boys' dependency scores decline more rapidly than do girls' dependency scores during late childhood (Golightly et al., 1970; Kagan & Moss, 1960). Gender differences in dependency remain relatively stable through adolescence, young adulthood, and middle adulthood (Chiriboga & Thurnher, 1980; Frank, Avery, & Laman, 1988; Mischel, 1970), with women continuing to show higher scores than men on self-report measures of dependency. Ultimately, however, gender differences in dependency diminish in later adulthood: Although both men and women show overall increases in self-reported dependency with increasing age, men show a more rapid increase in self-reported dependency than do women from middle to late adulthood (see Helson & Wink, 1992; Kalish, 1969).

In this context, it is important to note that aside from any age-related variations in overall level of dependency that may occur, studies confirm that the "object" of an individual's dependent strivings (i.e., the person toward whom dependent behaviors tend to be directed most readily) changes over time (see, e.g., Barry et al., 1965; Bauermeister, 1982; Birtchnell, 1988b; Caspi et al., 1989; Gewirtz, 1956b; Heathers, 1955b; Maccoby & Masters, 1970; Rosenthal, 1967; Sears, 1972; Sears et al., 1965; Takahashi, 1970). Specifically, young children tend to direct their dependent behavior toward parents (especially the primary caretaker), while in middle childhood teachers and other authority figures become important objects for the child's dependent strivings. As adolescence approaches, dependency is increasingly directed toward peers rather than toward figures of authority. Finally, in adulthood, dependent strivings are directed toward spouses, toward various pseudo-parental authority figures (e.g., employers, supervisors, physicians), and—to a lesser extent—toward peers, parents, and siblings.

Thus, as Ainsworth (1969) suggested, dependent behaviors that are first displayed in the child's relationship with the primary caretaker ultimately are exhibited in various other relationships. Clearly, the generalization of dependency from the infant–caretaker relationship to other "age-appropriate" relationships is caused by at least two factors: (1) changes in family structure and (2) societal pressures. As dependency on the primary caretaker of infancy becomes less and less feasible (and less and less appropriate), substitute caretakers are sought out by the dependent individual. In this context, Hoffman, (1984), Hoffman and Weiss (1987), and Rice (1992) have discussed in detail the negative consequences of strong parent-directed dependency stivings in adolescents and adults.

Not only does the object of an individual's dependency strivings change over time, but the way in which dependency is expressed also changes with increasing age. In light of societal norms regarding behaviors that are (and are not) permissible at different ages, this conclusion is hardly surprising. However, it is worth noting that in general, dependency-related behaviors during early childhood are manifested primarily via "demands" for physical comfort and contact (Sroufe, 1983; Sroufe et al., 1983). Subsequently, dependency is expressed via help-, reassurance-, and attention-seeking behaviors (see Caspi et al., 1989; Emmerich, 1966; Heathers, 1955b; Sears, 1963). With increasing age, dependency is increasingly displayed in indirect, "socially appropriate" ways (e.g., via conformity, compliance, and interpersonal yielding) and is expressed less and less via childlike attention-seeking behaviors (Fisher & Greenberg, 1985; Frank et al., 1988; Zirkel, 1992).

This may help to explain why global measures of dependency show substantially better stability over time (and across situation) than do more narrow situation- and person-specific indices of dependent behavior (see Maccoby & Masters, 1970; Mischel, 1970; Moskowitz, 1982). While an individual's level of dependency relative to others in his or her age cohort generally remains consistent over time, the specific behaviors that are used to express dependency strivings evolve as maturation occurs. Dependency-related behaviors that lead to positive outcomes at an early age may not yield the same benefits at later stages of development. Thus, dependent individuals learn to express dependency strivings in different ways at different times, attempting to select those behaviors that maximize the chances that they will obtain the nurturance, guidance, and support that they seek.

## Dependency and Sex Role

One of the most important determinants of the specific form that dependency strivings will take in boys and girls (and in men and women) is sex-role socialization. Traditional sex-role socialization practices lead men to express dependency needs indirectly, and lead women to express dependency needs in a more direct and overt manner (Maccoby & Jacklin, 1974; Mischel, 1970). Moreover, the causes of the increasing gender differences in self-reported dependency that begin to occur during late childhood may also lie in traditional sex-role socialization practices. As discussed in Chapter 1, boys are generally discouraged from expressing openly dependent feelings and needs, whereas girls have historically been encouraged to exhibit these feelings because passive, dependent behavior has traditionally been regarded as consonant with the female (i.e., "feminine") sex role. Thus, while projective tests and other "subtle" measures suggest that boys and girls (and men and women) have comparable underlying dependency needs, cultural factors serve to encourage the overt expression of these needs in women and to discourage the overt expression of these needs in men.

If men and women have comparable underlying dependency needs (as studies using projective measures of dependency suggest), but the overt expression of these needs is largely a function of sex-role socialization, then self-reported dependency should vary as a function of the degree to which men and women adopt traditional sex roles. To the degree that a woman views herself as departing from the traditional female sex role, she should be less willing to acknowledge dependency needs on self-report measures. Conversely, to the degree that a man regards himself as departing from the traditional male sex role, he should show higher levels of dependency on self-report tests. A number of studies have addressed this issue, directly or indirectly (Anderson, 1986; Birtchnell & Kennard, 1983; Cherniss, 1972; Chevron et al., 1978; Dempewolff, 1974; McClain, 1978; Ojha & Singh, 1985; Watson, Biderman, & Boyd, 1989; Welkowitz, Lish, & Bond, 1985; Zuroff, Moskowitz, Wielgus, Powers, & Franko, 1983).

Birtchnell and Kennard (1983) used a particularly inventive approach to examine the dependency–sex-role relationship. They compared the MMPI Dy scores of married women who reported that they and their spouse conformed to traditional sex roles (i.e., with the husband viewed as the "dominant" marriage partner) ($n$ of couples = 130) to the Dy scores of women who reported a reversal of traditional sex roles in their marriage (i.e., with the wife viewed as the dominant partner) ($n$ of couples = 46). As predicted, women who reported ascribing to the traditional marital role obtained significantly higher scores on the MMPI Dy scale than did women who reported a reversal of traditional sex roles in their marriage. Birtchnell and Kennard also found an inverse relationship between Dy scores and scores on the MMPI Do (dominance) scale in both male and female subjects in their study. Virtually identical results were obtained by Ojha and Singh (1985) in their investigation of dependency and marriage-role attitudes in Indian subjects.

The dependent women in Birtchnell and Kennard's (1983) sample also reported receiving inadequate amounts of affection from their husbands, while nondependent women reported receiving satisfactory amounts of affection. However, it is impossible to tell from these data whether high- and low-dependent women actually received different amounts of affection from their husbands, or whether high-and low-dependent women have different criterion levels for what constitutes an "adequate" amount of affection. Unfortunately, Birtchnell and Kennard did not examine the relationship between Dy score and perceived amount of affection received by their male subjects.

Zuroff and DeLorimier (1989) also assessed the relationship of dependency to perceptions of romantic partners, and obtained results that were generally consistent with those of Birtchnell and Kennard (1983). Subjects in Zuroff and DeLorimier's study were 66 undergraduate women who completed the DEQ dependency scale (Blatt et al., 1976) and provided descriptions of their "ideal" and "actual" romantic partners. Although dependency scores were unrelated to subjects' descriptions of actual romantic partners, a significant positive correlation ($r$ = .36) was found between dependency score and ratings of the ideal partner's need for intimacy. Dependent subjects desired a greater need for intimacy in their ideal romantic partners than did nondependent subjects (see also Birtchnell [1988b] for a discussion of some related findings).

Five studies have assessed directly the relationship of dependency to sex-role orientation (Anderson, 1986; Chevron et al., 1978; Watson et al., 1989; Welkowitz et al., 1985; Zuroff et al., 1983). These studies produced highly consistent findings. Table 3.2 summarizes the results of these five investigations. Three of the studies listed in Table 3.2 (i.e., those by Chevron et al., Welkowitz et al., and Zuroff et al.) used the DEQ dependency scale to assess level of dependency, whereas Anderson used Jones's (1957) Dependency Inventory, and Watson et al. used their own self-report dependency measure. In every study but one, sex-role orientation was assessed via the Bem (1974) Sex Role Inventory (BSRI). However, Chevron et al. used Broverman, Vogel, Broverman, Clarkson and Rosenkrantz's (1972) Sex Role Stereotype Questionnaire (SRSQ) to assess sex-role orientation.

As Table 3.2 shows, studies in this area generally obtained significant negative correlations between dependency and masculinity scores in both men and women.[7] Dependency–masculinity score correlations ranged from $-.02$ to $-.36$ for men, and from $-.11$ to $-.48$ for women, with the mean dependency–masculinity correlations being $-.23$ for men and $-.34$ for women. In contrast, these studies typically found a significant positive correlation between dependency and femininity scores in men but not in women. Dependency–femininity score correlations ranged from .09 to .52 for men, with the mean dependency–femininity correlation being .35. However, dependency–femininity score correlations for women ranged

**TABLE 3.2. Studies of Dependency and Sex-Role Orientation**

| | Dependency–sex-role correlation | | | |
| --- | --- | --- | --- | --- |
| | Masculinity scores | | Femininity scores | |
| Study | Men | Women | Men | Women |
| Anderson (1986) | $-.02$ | $-.34$ | .52 | $-.01$ |
| Chevron et al. (1978) | $-.36$ | $-.48$ | .42 | .07 |
| Watson et al. (1989) | $-.29$ | $-.29$ | .09 | .09 |
| Welkowitz et al. (1985) | $-.22$ | $-.11$ | .43 | .20 |
| Zuroff et al. (1983) | $-.27$ | $-.48$ | .27 | .11 |

*Note.* Data for the Watson et al. (1989) study were not reported separately for men and women. Watson et al. reported no sex differences in dependency–sex-role orientation correlations and therefore presented pooled data only.

from −.01 to .20, and the mean dependency–femininity score correlation for women was only .09 (although it must be noted that four of the five dependency–femininity correlations obtained in women were in the predicted direction). In short, studies conducted to date confirm that there is a significant relationship between level of dependency and self-reports of sex-role orientation, but overall, the relationship of dependency to masculinity scores is somewhat stronger than is the relationship of dependency to femininity scores.

Along slightly different lines, several studies have examined the relationship between dependency and feminist attitudes in women (e.g., Cherniss, 1972; Dempewolff, 1974; McClain, 1978). Insofar as feminism in women can be viewed as a departure from the traditional female sex role, these investigations provide further information regarding the dependency–sex-role relationship. These studies all used self-report measures of both dependency and feminism. In each of these studies, high feminism scores were associated with lower dependency scores in women.

McClain's (1978) study illustrates the general pattern of results obtained in these investigations. McClain selected high- and low-feminism undergraduate women based on scores on a 40-item questionnaire of feminist ideology, and compared the scores of high- and low-feminism subjects on a variety of dependency measures, including the 16PF Dependence–Independence scale (Cattell, 1966). As predicted, feminist women obtained significantly lower dependency scores than did nonfeminist women on every dependency scale. Virtually identical results were obtained by Dempewolff (1974). Similar results were also obtained by Cherniss (1972), although the relatively unsystematic data collection and data-analytic procedures used by Cherniss limit the degree to which strong conclusions can be drawn from his investigation.

The results of studies assessing the relationship of dependency to sex-role orientation clearly support the hypothesis that the overt expression of dependency needs in both men and women is a function of the degree to which subjects ascribe to traditional sex roles. Unfortunately, studies in this area do not address the question of whether men and women who show "masculine" characteristics actually perceive themselves as having low levels of dependency needs or instead perceive themselves as having strong dependency needs but are unwilling to acknowledge these needs on self-report measures. Furthermore, these studies do not provide information regarding the causal relationship between dependency and sex role. It is possible that departure from the traditional sex role influences the overt expression of dependency needs in men and women. However, an equally tenable interpretation of these findings is that level of dependency somehow plays a role in determining sex-role characteristics in adults. A longitudinal study of the dependency–sex-role relationship would begin to address this issue.

## NOTES

1. It is worth noting that several studies have also examined the relationship between birth order and dependency, testing the hypothesis that first-born and only children would show significantly higher dependency levels than would later-born children (see Masling, Weiss, & Rothchild [1968] for a detailed discussion of this hypothesis). These investigations produced inconsistent findings, with two studies obtaining the predicted dependency–birth order relationship (Schachter, 1959; Sears et al., 1957), three studies obtaining the opposite results (i.e., higher dependency scores in later-born children than in first-born children) (Feldman, 1978; Masling et al., 1968; Rim, 1981), and one study obtaining nonsignificant results (Vats, 1986).

2. Throughout this book I use the term *nondependent* rather than *independent* to refer to individuals who obtain low scores on various dependency measures. I use this term because the majority of dependency measures are structured in such a way that a low score merely indicates an absence of dependent thoughts, feelings, and/or behaviors. However, a low score on most dependency measures does not necessarily indicate a high degree of independence. Thus, the control subjects to whom dependent persons are compared are most accurately described as nondependent—rather than independent—persons.

3. In this context, it is worth noting that at least three studies have found a relationship between socioeconomic status (SES) and dependency, with children from low-SES backgrounds showing higher levels of dependency than children from middle- and high-SES families (Bhogle, 1983; Drake, Adler, & Vaillant, 1988; Fu et al., 1984). These results are consistent with the well-established finding that low-SES parents tend to utilize more authoritarian parenting practices than do middle- and high-SES parents (see Maccoby, 1980). Thus, these results provide additional indirect support for a relationship between authoritarian parenting and dependency.

4. Because overprotective and authoritarian parenting practices both lead to high levels of dependency in children, I tried to find a convenient term under which both parenting styles could be subsumed. Two terms presented themselves: *dependency-fostering* parenting and *dependogenic* parenting (the latter term being a derivative of Bateson, Jackson, Haley, & Weakland's [1956] *schizophrenogenic* parent). However, the first term didn't seem very informative, and the second term is kind of awkward. Thus, for the remainder of the book, I will continue to refer to "overprotective, authoritarian parenting practices." When I use this term, I am referring to parents who show high levels of *either or both* of these traits.

5. Although a few studies in this area reported significant parent gender × child gender interactions when assessing the effects of parenting style on the development of children's dependency (e.g., Baumrind, 1967, 1971; Sears, 1963; Sears et al., 1965), the majority of investigations found that parental overprotectiveness and authoritarianism have similar effects on boys' and girls' dependency levels regardless of whether parenting style ratings are taken from the mother, the father, or both parents. Overall, global ratings of parenting style predict children's dependency levels at least as well as do more specific ratings of maternal and paternal parenting practices.

6. Interestingly, a similar pattern seems to characterize studies of dependency in children that use rating scales versus direct behavioral observations. As Yeger and Miezitis (1985) noted: "[Although] sex differences [in dependency] tend to appear in studies using rating scales of pupils' behavior . . . they appear less frequently in studies using direct behavioral observation. Since rating scales are subject to response sets and other sorts of biases on the part of the rater, this is strong evidence that raters in general, and teachers in particular, are subject to a stereotyped evaluation of the sexes" (p. 460). Similar conclusions were drawn by Maccoby and Jacklin (1974) following their extensive review of research on gender differences in development.

7. Mussen (1961) also obtained a significant negative correlation ($r = -.30$) between masculinity scores and dependency scores in a sample of adolscent boys. Because the validity of the masculinity scale used in this study was questionable, I did not include Mussen's data in Table 3.2. It is worth noting, however, that Mussen's findings are consistent with those reported in other studies of the dependency–masculinity relationship.

# *Interpersonal Correlates of Dependency*

Theoretical disputes regarding the etiology and development of dependency notwithstanding, it is clear that dependency is, above all, a social phenomenon. The studies reviewed in Chapter 3 leave little doubt that individual differences in dependency can be traced to early social interactions. Initially, these interactions take place within the infant–caretaker dyad. Subsequently, social learning that takes place within the family influences the development of dependency. Ultimately, interactions with peers, teachers, and other important figures further influence the ways in which dependency needs are expressed. Given the social roots of dependency, it is hardly surprising to learn that dependency affects the interpersonal behavior of children and adults in predictable ways. Regardless of whether one favors the psychoanalytic model, the social learning model, or some other theoretical framework, it seems that—as far as dependency is concerned—early social interactions predict the nature of later social interactions.

In this chapter I review empirical studies that examine the effects of dependency on social behavior. These studies can be divided into three categories: (1) studies of suggestibility, yielding, and compliance; (2) studies of help-seeking behavior, affiliative tendencies, and sensitivity to interpersonal cues; and (3) studies of performance anxiety and response to evaluation by figures of authority.

## DEPENDENCY, SUGGESTIBILITY, YIELDING, AND COMPLIANCE

The dependent person is hypothesized to be highly motivated to please other people in order to obtain nurturance and support (Millon, 1981; Tripathi, 1982). This should lead the dependent person to minimize interpersonal conflict whenever possible and to engage in behaviors that promote good relationships with peers and figures of authority. Thus, dependency should be associated with suggestibility, interpersonal yielding, and compliance with others' requests, demands, and expectations. Each of these hypothesized relationships has been examined empirically.

## Dependency and Suggestibility

One of the first investigations in this area was conducted by Zuckerman and Grosz (1958), who examined the relationship between dependency (assessed via the TAT and EPPS) and hypnotic suggestibility in a mixed-sex undergraduate sample. As predicted, dependent subjects were more more receptive to hypnotic suggestions than were nondependent subjects. One would expect, based on these results, that dependent subjects would also be more easily hypnotized than would nondependent subjects. Unfortunately, however, Zuckerman and Grosz did not examine directly the relationship between dependency and hypnotizability in this investigation.

Zuckerman and Grosz's (1958) results were interesting, but their study was really a pilot investigation, not a full-scale experiment. A somewhat more sophisticated (and extensive) study of the dependency–suggestibility relationship was conducted by Jakubczak and Walters (1959), who investigated the relationship between these variables in a sample of 24 9-year-old boys. Subjects in this study were divided into high- and low-dependent groups based on responses to a projective dependency measure. Each subject then participated in a standard autokinetic effect experiment, with erroneous judgments regarding the movement of a stationary light source provided by either a high-status confederate (i.e., an adult male) or a same-sex peer. A number of interesting findings emerged from Jakubczak and Walters's study, but two results in particular are noteworthy in the present context. First, there was a main effect of subject dependency on susceptibility to the autokinetic effect: Dependent subjects were more susceptible than nondependent subjects to the effect, regardless of the status of the confederate. Second, subject dependency and confederate status interacted to predict susceptibility to the autokinetic effect: The influence of confederate status on susceptibility to the effect was significantly greater for dependent than nondependent subjects.

Jakubczak and Walters's (1959) results not only suggest that dependency is associated with increased suggestibility in laboratory settings, but further indicate that this effect is particularly pronounced when the source of information is a high-status person rather than a peer. The latter result (i.e., dependent persons' greater susceptibility to interpersonal influence from high-status than low-status individuals), which was demonstrated for the first time in Jakubczak and Walters's experiment, turns out to be a very significant finding. As the ensuing review of the social literature will show, this pattern of results emerges in a variety of areas and has important implications for understanding and predicting the behavior of dependent persons in social settings.

Jakubczak and Walters's (1959) findings were eventually replicated and extended by Tribich and Messer (1974), who selected dependent and non-dependent undergraduate male subjects according to scores on Blum's (1949) Blacky test. Consistent with Jakubczak and Walters's earlier results, Tribich and Messer found enhanced susceptibility to the autokinetic effect in dependent subjects relative to nondependent subjects. Furthermore, high-status confederates again had a significantly greater influence on dependent subjects' judgments than did low-status confederates, but confederate status did not produce differential effects on the judgments made by nondependent subjects.

Finally, using a different paradigm (ratings of slogan credibility), subject sample (Indian college students), and measure of dependency (Sinha's [1968] DP scale), Ojha (1972) obtained results that were very similar to those reported by Jakubczak and Walters (1959) and Tribich and Messer (1974). Ojha found that dependent subjects of both sexes rated a series of political slogans as more credible and convincing when they were associated with high-prestige individuals than when they were associated with low-prestige persons. However, as predicted, no effects of source prestige on slogan credibility were found for the nondependent subjects in Ojha's sample.

## Dependency and Yielding

Studies of dependency and interpersonal yielding are generally consistent with findings regarding the dependency–suggestibility relationship, and provide further evidence supporting the hypothesis that the behavior of dependent individuals is more strongly affected by high-status than low-status persons. Two experiments investigated the dependency–yielding relationship using an Asch (1956) conformity paradigm. First, Kagan and Mussen (1956) found that high TAT dependency scores were associated with increased yielding to the majority opinion in an Asch-type experiment where male subjects made judgments regarding the length of lines, with confederate subjects providing erroneous opinions before the actual subject offered his judgment. Similarly, Masling, Weiss, and Rothschild (1968) found that dependent male subjects (selected according to scores on Masling et al.'s [1967] ROD scale) were more likely than nondependent subjects to acquiesce to the opinions of confederates when estimating the number of clicking sounds in a modified Asch-type conformity experiment.

One study in this area (Bornstein, Masling, & Poynton, 1987) obtained the opposite results (i.e., an inverse relationship between dependency and yielding). In Bornstein et al.'s experiment, dependent and nondependent male undergraduates were selected according to scores on Masling et al.'s (1967) ROD scale. Subjects were informed that they were taking part in a study of the decision-making process. Pairs consisting of one dependent and one nondependent subject were constructed, and subjects were asked individually to attempt to determine the gender of 10 poets, provided only with brief poem excerpts. The experimenter then compared the guesses of the two members of each subject pair, and selected three poems on which the subjects had disagreed. The experimenter asked the two subjects to discuss these three poems for 10 minutes and to resolve their disagreement and reach a consensus decision regarding the gender of the three poets.

Bornstein et al. (1987) found that dependent subjects were significantly less likely than nondependent subjects to change their initial opinions: In 35 of 50 dyads (70%), the nondependent subject yielded to the opinion of the dependent subject on the majority of poems. At first, this finding seems counterintuitive and inconsistent with earlier studies of dependency and yielding. However, postexperiment interviews revealed that dependent subjects were particularly concerned with making a good impression on the experimenter. The majority of dependent subjects cited this as the primary reason that they did not change their initial opinions. Because the subjects' initial opinions were known to the experimenter (unlike an Asch-type experiment, where the subject is not required to alter an initial "public" opinion), changing the initial opinion involved the risk that the experimenter would regard the subject in a negative way.

Thus, when confronted with choosing between impressing a figure of authority (the experimenter) or getting along with a peer (the other subject), dependent individuals opted to stand by their initial opinion and thereby impress the authority figure. In this respect, Bornstein et al.'s (1987) results are consistent with earlier findings regarding the dependency–suggestibility relationship, which indicated that dependent individuals are more strongly influenced by the opinions of authority figures than by the opinions of peers (Jakubczak & Walters, 1959; Ojha, 1972; Tribich & Messer, 1974).

## Dependency and Compliance

A number of laboratory and field studies have investigated the relationship of dependency to compliance with the demands and expectations of others. In most of these investigations, compliant behavior was examined directly (Agrawal & Rai, 1988; Bornstein & Masling, 1985; Gorton, 1975; Griffith, 1991; Levitt, Lubin, & Zuckerman, 1962; Masling, O'Neill, & Jayne, 1981; Weiss, 1969), although in one study self-reports of compliance were assessed (Biaggio, Godwin, & Baldwin, 1984).

Three general strategies have been used to assess compliant behavior in studies of the dependency–compliance link. In the laboratory, researchers have examined the relationship of level of dependency to (1) persistence in frustrating puzzle-solving tasks and (2) compliance with the perceived expectations of the experimenter. In field studies, researchers have operationalized compliance in terms of willingness to serve as experimental subjects under various conditions.

Agrawal and Rai's (1988) investigation used the first of these three strategies. Agrawal and Rai divided a mixed-sex sample of 120 undergraduate subjects into high-, moderate-, and low-dependent groups according to scores on Sinha's (1968) DP scale. They then asked subjects to attempt to solve a series of four puzzles as quickly as possible. The first two puzzles were soluble, but the second two were insoluble. Subjects were instructed to continue working on the puzzles until they had solved all four; the dependent measure of compliance used in this study was the amount of time that subjects persisted in attempting to solve the two insoluble puzzles. As predicted, Agrawal and Rai found a significant positive relationship between DP score and persistence in the puzzle-solving task, with high-DP subjects spending the longest amount of time on the task, followed by moderate-DP subjects. Low-DP subjects spent significantly less time attempting to solve the insoluble puzzles than did the high- or moderate-DP subjects.

Using a very different procedure, measure of compliance, and measure of dependency, Weiss (1969) obtained results generally consistent with those of Agrawal and Rai (1988). Weiss selected dependent and nondependent undergraduate subjects according to scores on the Blacky test and informed the subjects that they were participating in a study of perceptual processes in normal college students. She then presented a series of slides with different numbers of dots randomly placed and asked the subjects to estimate the number of dots on each slide. Half the subjects were told that "college students like you typically overestimate the number of dots on these slides," and half were told that "college students like you typically underestimate the number of dots on these slides."

As predicted, Weiss (1969) found that dependent subjects' estimates were more strongly influenced by the experimenter's "expectations" than were nondependent subjects' estimates: Dependent subjects over- or underestimated the number of dots in accordance with the perceived expectations of the experimenter, while nondependent subjects showed relatively little compliance with the experimenter's expectations. An important strength of this study was Weiss's use of a "covert" compliance measure. In contrast to Agrawal and Rai's (1988) experiment, wherein subjects were explicitly instructed to persist in the problem-solving task that served as the dependent measure of compliance, in Weiss's experiment subjects never received explicit instructions regarding how to respond. The fact that Weiss obtained results consistent with those of Agrawal and Rai suggests that dependent subjects in psychology experiments actively search for cues to tell them what the experimenter wants them to do and then proceed to comply with these perceived expectations.

Studies by Masling et al. (1981) and Bornstein and Masling (1985) provide additional support for the hypothesized dependency–compliance link. However, these studies examined the dependency–compliance relationship in a more naturalistic setting: the classroom. In these investigations, ROD scores (Masling et al., 1967) were obtained from samples of introductory psychology students who were required to participate in several psychology experiments during the course of a semester in order to fulfill the introductory psychology research participation requirement. Each subject's ROD scores were then compared to the week in the semester that he or she completed the required experiments. Masling et al. (1981) and Bornstein and Masling (1985) hypothesized that dependent subjects would complete the research participation requirement earlier in the semester than would nondependent subjects, because dependent subjects should be more concerned than nondependent subjects with pleasing their psychology professor by complying with the professor's request that they complete their research requirement in a timely manner. Strong support for this hypothesis was obtained. In both experiments, there was a significant inverse relationship between ROD score and week in the semester at which the research participation requirement was completed.

Similarly, Levitt et al. (1962) found that Rorschach dependency scores predicted likelihood of volunteering to participate in an experiment on hypnotizability in two separate samples of female nursing students. These findings are particularly compelling because (1) they were obtained in two independent subject samples and (2) no payment or course credit was offered to the study volunteers. Thus, dependency not only predicts latency of volunteering to serve as experimental subjects among introductory psychology students (as the findings of Masling et al. [1981] and Bornstein & Masling [1985] indicate), but also predicts likelihood of volunteering to participate in experiments when no payment or rewards are offered.[1]

The only study in this area that assessed self-reported compliance rather than actual compliant behavior is also the only study that failed to find the predicted dependency–compliance relationship. Biaggio et al. (1984) selected groups of dependent and nondependent undergraduates based on scores on Navran's (1954) MMPI Dy scale. They then had subjects read a series of vignettes describing interpersonal interactions in which one person made an unreasonable demand on another person (e.g., an employee asks a coworker to stay late at work and complete his tasks so that the employee can leave work early). Subjects were asked to make three 7-point ratings for each vignette: (1) the degree to which they would comply with the request if it was made to them; (2) the amount of anger that they would feel toward the requester; and (3) the amount of sympathy that they would feel for the requester.

Biaggio et al. (1984) found no differences between dependent and nondependent subjects on any rating dimension. They attributed their nonsignificant findings to the artificiality of the design of this experiment, and it is clear that—as Biaggio et al. (1984) suggest—the use of self-report rather than behavioral measures of compliance might well have played a role in producing the negative results obtained in this study. However, it is also worth noting, in the context of the present review, that dependent subjects would not have been expected to report increased compliance with the excessive demands described in Biaggio et al.'s (1984) vignettes. As studies by Bornstein et al. (1987) and others demonstrated, dependent subjects are more concerned with pleasing figures of authority than with accommodating the demands of peers. In the Biaggio et al. (1984) study, acquiescence to unreasonable demands from a peer might well be interpreted by dependent subjects as reflecting negatively on them. For example, acquiescing to such demands might cause the experimenter to view the subject as weak or "wishy-washy." Thus, even if the dependent subjects wanted to comply more strongly than did the nondependent subjects in Biaggio et al.'s (1984) experiment (and it is not at all clear from these data that that is the case), self-presentation needs might well have obviated any dependency effects that did in fact exist.

Overall, studies of suggestibility, yielding, and compliance have produced strong, consistent findings that may be summarized as follows. First, dependency is associated with a general tendency to be influenced by the opinions of others, to yield to others in interpersonal transactions, and to comply with others' expectations and demands. However, when placed in a position where he or she must choose between getting along with a peer or pleasing a figure of authority, the dependent individual will typically opt for pleasing the authority figure. In a sense, this pattern of results is not surprising: Given the dependent person's concern with being nurtured and supported by others, it is clear that choosing to please authority figures rather than peers simply reflects the dependent person's attempt to maximize gain, that is, to curry favor with the individual most likely to be able to offer the guidance, support, and protection that the dependent person seeks.

The finding that dependent individuals are able to direct their dependency-related behaviors toward different persons in different contexts stands in stark contrast to findings from studies of attachment behaviors in children, adolescents, and adults. In these investigations, there is relatively little variability in the "object" of an individual's attachment-related behaviors, at least in the short term (Ainsworth, 1972, 1989; Maccoby &

Masters, 1970). In other words, as noted in Chapter 1, attachment behaviors are "person specific." In contrast, the studies reviewed in this section suggest that dependency-related behaviors are "nonspecific" insofar as they are directed toward different persons at different times. Thus, these findings are consistent with the suggestions of Gewirtz (1956b), Ainsworth (1972) and others, who hypothesized that while an individual's level of dependency may be stable over time, the persons toward whom dependency-related behaviors will be directed change over time and across situation (see Chapter 3 for a detailed discussion of this issue).

## DEPENDENCY, HELP SEEKING, INTERPERSONAL SENSITIVITY, AND AFFILIATION

The results of studies examining the relationship of dependency to suggestibility, yielding, and compliance confirm that dependent persons often assume a passive role in interpersonal interactions, allowing others to take the lead in structuring the interaction and determining the outcome of the situation. These results further indicate that the dependent person is inclined to seek the guidance of others—especially figures of authority—when confronted with a task or problem. Thus, findings regarding the dependency–suggestibility, dependency–yielding, and dependency–compliance relationships lead to several additional hypotheses regarding the interpersonal correlates of dependency.

First, these findings suggest that dependent persons should show elevated rates of help-seeking behaviors in a variety of situations and settings (see Fisher & Greenberg [1985] for a detailed discussion of this hypothesis). Several studies have examined directly the dependency–help-seeking relationship in children and adults (Bernardin & Jessor, 1957; Diener, 1967; Flanders, Anderson, & Amidon, 1961; Shilkret & Masling, 1981; Sinha & Pandey, 1972; Sroufe et al., 1983).

Second, if obtaining support from others is important to the dependent person, dependency should be associated with sensitivity to interpersonal cues: To the extent that dependent individuals are able to infer accurately the attitudes, beliefs, and feelings of others, they should be better able to obtain the help and support that they desire. In this context, researchers have examined the relationship between dependency and interpersonal sensitivity in both laboratory (Masling, O'Neill, & Katkin, 1982; Wilson & Shantz, 1977) and field settings (Masling, Johnson, & Saturansky, 1974).

Finally, if obtaining support from others is important to the dependent person, dependency should be associated with affiliative tendencies. Several studies have assessed the relationship of dependency to various indirect measures of affiliation (Burton, McGregor, & Berry, 1979; Exline & Messick, 1967; Juni et al., 1979; Keinan & Hobfoll, 1989; Libby & Yanklevich, 1973; Masling, Price, Goldband, & Katkin, 1981; Shilkret & Masling, 1981; Simpson & Gangestad, 1991; Sroufe et al., 1983). These studies all tested the hypothesis that dependency is associated with a desire to be close to others, especially when the dependent person feels anxious or threatened.

## Dependency and Help Seeking

Early studies of dependency and help seeking utilized male subjects and male experimenters only and produced highly consistent results. In the first of these investigations, Bernardin and Jessor (1957) found that dependent male subjects exhibited significantly more help-seeking behavior than did nondependent male subjects in a laboratory problem-solving situation. The measure of help seeking used by Bernardin and Jessor was the number of times that the subject asked a male experimenter for help while attempting to solve jigsaw puzzles. Bernardin and Jessor found that dependent subjects asked for help nearly four times as often as did nondependent subjects: The mean number of requests for help made by dependent subjects was 3.50, while the mean number of requests made by nondependent subjects was 0.95. It is worth noting, parenthetically, that dependent subjects also asked for reassurance significantly more often than did nondependent subjects: Dependent subjects sought reassurance from the experimenter an average of 10.90 times, while nondependent subjects sought reassurance only 1.45 times (nearly an eightfold difference).

Diener (1967) used the same procedure and experimental task as did Bernardin and Jessor (1957). Although Diener obtained a nonsignificant correlation ($r = .24$) between dependency and help-seeking scores in his sample of male psychiatric inpatients, the dependency–help-seeking relationship in Diener's study was in the predicted direction. Using a somewhat different experimental design, Sinha and Pandey (1972) found a significant positive correlation ($r = .42$) between DP score (Sinha, 1968) and the number of times that a subject requested help from the experimenter during a laboratory problem-solving task similar to that used by Bernardin and Jessor and Diener. Cairns (1961) also found a significant positive relationship ($r = .59$) between level of dependency and the number of times that a subject asked the experimenter for help during a puzzle-solving task.[2]

Along slightly different lines, Flanders et al. (1961) examined the relationship between dependency and help-seeking behavior in the classroom. In this study, a mixed-sex sample of elementary school students was classified into dependent and nondependent groups based on scores on a self-report measure of interpersonal dependency. Observational measures of dependent behavior in the classroom were then collected for each child. Dependent children of both sexes asked the teacher for help more frequently than did nondependent children, and sought approval and positive feedback from the teacher more frequently than did nondependent children. Virtually identical results were obtained by Beller (1959), who assessed the dependency–help-seeking relationship in a mixed-sex sample of preschool and nursery school children. Highly similar results were also obtained by Sroufe et al. (1983) in a mixed-sex sample of 40 nursery school children. The findings obtained by Flanders et al. (1961), Beller (1959), and Sroufe et al. (1983) in classroom settings parallel those obtained by Bernardin and Jessor (1958) and others in more structured laboratory situations (see also Yasunaga [1985] for similar findings regarding the dependency–help-seeking relationship in Japanese schoolchildren).

Only Shilkret and Masling (1981) assessed directly the effects of subject and experimenter gender on the dependency–help-seeking relationship. Shilkret and Masling asked 80 undergraduate subjects (40 women and 40 men) to solve a series of difficult puzzles (e.g., anagrams, jigsaw puzzles), with the caveat that they could ask the experimenter for help if they felt that they needed assistance at any time during the experiment. Half the subjects were assigned a male experimenter and half were assigned a female experimenter. Prior to participating in the puzzle-solving task, subjects had been divided into high- and low-dependent groups based on scores on Masling et al.'s (1967) ROD scale. The measure of help-seeking behavior used in Shilkret and Masling's study was the number of times that the subject asked the experimenter for help.

In three of four comparisons in Shilkret and Masling's (1981) experiment, the predicted positive relationship between dependency and help seeking was obtained. Dependent male subjects asked for help more frequently than did nondependent male subjects, regardless of the gender of the experimenter. However, dependent female subjects asked for help more frequently than did nondependent females only when a female experimenter was present; the predicted pattern of results was not found for female subjects with male experimenters. Shilkret and Masling suggested that the sexual connotations of a female subject asking a male authority figure for help may have obviated any dependency-related differences in help-seeking behavior.

Taken together, the results obtained in studies of dependency and help seeking are consistent with the hypothesis that dependent individuals ask for guidance and assistance from others more often than do nondependent individuals. However, the results of Shilkret and Masling's (1981) experiment further indicate that subject and experimenter gender may interact to determine the likelihood that a dependent subject will ask for help in the laboratory setting. Clearly, further research is needed to assess the generalizability of this result to nonlaboratory settings. In addition, research is needed to determine whether the dependency–help-seeking relationship is exhibited with peers as well as figures of authority. In all studies conducted to date examining the dependency–help-seeking relationship, the potential helper was an authority figure (i.e., a teacher or experimenter), and it is not clear from these studies whether similar behaviors would be exhibited by dependent individuals when peers—rather than authority figures—are potential helpers.

## Dependency and Interpersonal Sensitivity

In one of the most inventive and cleverly designed studies of the dependency–interpersonal sensitivity relationship, Masling et al. (1982) investigated whether dependent individuals would be more sensitive than nondependent individuals to warm versus cold treatment by a confederate. In this experiment, undergraduate male subjects were divided into dependent and nondependent groups based on scores on Masling et al.'s (1967) ROD scale. They were informed that they were taking part in a study of "how people get to know each other." Subjects then interacted for 10 minutes with a male confederate who treated them either in a warm, friendly manner or in a cold, distant manner. Subjects' electrodermal responses (EDRs) were recorded before, during, and after the interaction period.

Masling et al. (1982) found that as hypothesized, dependent subjects responded differentially to warm versus cold treatment by the confederate: Dependent subjects' EDRs increased significantly from baseline (preinteraction) to postconversation period only in the "cold" condition. In the "warm" condition, dependent subjects' EDRs remained unchanged from baseline to postconversation period. In contrast, nondependent subjects showed no differential responding to warm versus cold treatment by the confederate. Although this experiment demonstrated that dependent subjects respond differentially to warm versus cold treatment by a peer, the results of this study also raise an interesting question. The design of Masling et al.'s (1982) experiment was such that it is impossible to tell from their results whether subjects were consciously aware of the confederate's treatment of them (and if so, whether they would have been willing to acknowledge this if asked). Thus, one wonders whether self-report measures would have produced results similar to those obtained via the EDR measures that were used in this experiment.

An earlier study by Masling et al. (1974) suggested that under certain conditions, dependent individuals are more accurate social perceivers than are nondependent individuals. Two experiments comprised this study. In the first, a mixed-sex sample of undergraduates was divided into dependent and nondependent groups based on scores on Masling et al.'s (1967) ROD scale. Each subject was then randomly paired with another subject, and the two members of each dyad were given 15 minutes to "get acquainted" with each other. Following the conversations, subjects individually completed a questionnaire that asked about their beliefs, attitudes, and personal characteristics. Finally, each subject was given an identical questionnaire and was asked to complete it as he or she thought that his or her partner would. The measure of interpersonal sensitivity in this study was the concordance of the subject's guesses with the partner's self-ratings. Masling et al. (1974) obtained mixed results in this experiment. Dependent males were better predictors of their male partners' responses than were nondependent males. However, no differences in predictive accuracy were found for dependent versus nondependent females, nor were dependent subjects of either sex more accurate predictors than nondependent subjects in mixed-sex dyads.

Masling et al. (1974) then conducted a more naturalistic follow-up study to test the replicability and generalizability of their initial results. In the follow-up study, a similar methodology was employed except that (1) Peace Corps volunteers were used instead of undergraduates and (2) subjects attempted to guess the questionnaire responses of their roommates rather than attempting to guess the responses of an individual that they had known for only 15 minutes. As in the first study, dependent male subjects were significantly more accurate than nondependent males in their inferences regarding roommates' attitudes, beliefs, and personal characteristics. However, no effect of dependency on the accuracy of female subjects' inferences was found.

Juni and Semel (1982) performed a modified replication of Masling et al.'s (1974) experiment. In Juni and Semel's study, undergraduate students participating in a psychology seminar were asked to make judgments regarding the attitudes, interests, and personal beliefs of the female seminar leader after a brief (i.e., 10-minute) discussion period. In contrast to Masling et al.'s (1974) results, Juni and Semel found that dependency predicted the accuracy of students' descriptions of the discussion leader for female subjects only: The correlation between ROD score and accuracy of descriptions was .44 for women and $-.08$ for men.

Only one study (Wilson & Shantz, 1977) examined the relationship between dependency and interpersonal sensitivity in children. In this study, 25 nursery school children were individually rated for level of dependency by their nursery school teacher. Each child then completed a series of role-taking tasks in which his or her ability to infer accurately the thoughts and feelings of a fictional target person was assessed (see Wilson & Shantz [1977] for a detailed description of the procedures and scoring of the role-taking task). Consistent with findings regarding dependency and interpersonal sensitivity in adults, Wilson and Shantz found a significant positive correlation between dependency score and score on the role-taking task in their child subjects ($r$ = .53), with dependent children showing better role-taking ability than nondependent children.

Thus, research conducted to date generally supports the hypothesis that dependency is associated with interpersonal sensitivity in both children and adults. However, two qualifications of this conclusion warrant mention. First, with the exception of Juni and Semel's (1982) results, the dependency–interpersonal sensitivity relationship in adults is generally stronger for men than for women. Second, in every sample examined, the accuracy of cross-gender predictions has been unrelated to dependency. This latter result is not too surprising, in light of the fact that our perceptions of—and inferences regarding—opposite-sex people are likely to be strongly influenced by a number of factors unrelated to level of dependency (e.g., degree of sexual attraction).

## Dependency and Affiliative Behavior

Unfortunately, although there have been a number of studies of dependency and affiliative tendencies, none of the dependent variables used in these investigations is a direct measure of need for affiliation. To date, researchers have used five different types of dependent variables in these studies. Simpson and Gangestad (1991) examined degree of commitment to a romantic relationship; Masling et al. (1981) assessed autonomic arousal in social isolation; Keinan and Hobfoll (1989) assessed state anxiety during childbirth; several studies (Hollender, Luborsky, & Harvey, 1970; Juni et al., 1979; Sroufe et al., 1983) assessed physical touching; and several studies (Burton et al., 1979; Exline & Messick, 1967; Libby & Yanklevich, 1973; Shilkret & Masling, 1981) investigated the amount of eye contact engaged in by dependent versus nondependent subjects. I will briefly review studies in these five areas.

Simpson and Gangestad (1991) hypothesized that dependency would be associated with increased commitment in romantic relationships because the dependent person is particularly concerned with maintaining close ties to supportive, nurturing figures. Although Simpson and Gangestad's investigation was not concerned with affiliative tendencies per se, the results of this study nonetheless have important implications for the dependency–affiliation relationship. Two hundred forty-one unmarried monogamous couples participated in the study. Each subject provided three pieces of information: (1) a self-report of level of dependency, using Bersheid and Fei's (1977) dependency scale; (2) a rating of his or her degree of commitment to the relationship; and (3) an estimate of his or her partner's degree of commitment to the relationship.

Two noteworthy findings emerged from this investigation. First, there was a significant positive correlation between level of dependency and degree of commitment to the relationship in both men ($r = .59$) and women ($r = .49$). Second, there was a significant positive correlation between level of dependency and estimates of the partner's degree of commitment to the relationship in men ($r = .28$) and in women ($r = .29$). These results suggest not only that dependency is associated with increased commitment in romantic relationships, but also that level of dependency predicts subjects' perceptions of their partner's commitment to the relationship. The finding that dependency is associated with increased commitment in romantic relationships provides indirect support for the hypothesis that dependency is associated with affiliative tendencies. This result also echoes Kagan and Moss's (1960) finding that childhood dependency levels predict self-reports of the degree to which subjects view themselves as dependent on their spouses or romantic partners at ages 20–29 (see also Caspi et al. [1989] for a discussion of childhood dependency as a predictor of marital commitment and stability).

There are at least two possible explanations for Simpson and Gangestad's (1991) finding that level of dependency predicts subjects' perceptions of their romantic partner's degree of commitment to the relationship. The first (optimistic) interpretation of this result is that dependent individuals seek out romantic partners who show strong commitment to the relationship. If this is true, dependent people are able to identify (and develop relationships with) committed romantic partners—individuals who are likely to gratify the dependent person's need for nurturance and support. The second (less optimistic) interpretation of this result is that there is no relationship between level of dependency and the degree of commitment of one's romantic partner, but that dependent individuals are motivated to perceive their partners as being highly committed to the relationship. This latter interpretation of Simpson and Gangestad's findings would imply that dependent persons display a kind of self-serving bias (i.e., distortion) in perceptions of their romantic partners, perceiving greater commitment in the partner than actually exists.

If this should turn out to be the case, we must conclude that dependency influences interpersonal perception in two distinct ways. First, as Masling et al. (1974; Masling, Schiffner, & Shenfeld, 1980) and others have demonstrated, dependency is associated with sensitivity to interpersonal cues, at least with respect to relatively neutral information such as a roommate's or therapist's attitudes and personal beliefs. However, if the latter interpretation of Simpson and Gangestad's (1991) finding is correct, this would suggest that the dependent person is a particularly biased perceiver of self-referent information. Additional studies are needed to examine more closely the factors that underlie the observed relationship between level of dependency and perceptions of romantic partners' degree of commitment.

Masling, Price, Goldband, and Katkin (1981) used a different approach to examine the dependency—affiliation relationship. They divided a sample of undergraduate males into dependent and nondependent groups based on the subjects' ROD scores. Masling et al. then placed each subject in a soundproof chamber for 40 minutes under one of two conditions. Half the subjects were alone for the 40-minute period, and the remaining subjects were seated alongside a male confederate who was instructed to behave in a neutral manner (i.e., to act neither warm nor cold) toward the subject. The subjects (and confederates) were asked to complete several clerical tasks (e.g., checking phone numbers from a directory) during the experiment. Subjects' EDRs were recorded throughout the 40-minute period. Masling et al. hypothesized that dependent subjects would show greater arousal in the "alone" condition than in the "together" condition in this experiment, while nondependent subjects would show no differential responding in the two conditions. Strong support was obtained for this hypothesis, with dependent subjects showing significantly greater electrodermal responding in the "alone" than in the "together" condition and nondependent subjects showing comparable levels of responding in the two conditions.

Using a very different procedure, subject sample, and measure of anxiety, Keinan and Hobfoll (1989) obtained results remarkably similar to those of Masling, Price, Goldband, and Katkin (1981). In Keinan and Hobfoll's study, 67 pregnant Israeli women were divided into dependent and nondependent groups based on their scores on a self-report measure of interpersonal dependency. Twelve hours postdelivery, each woman reported whether her husband had been present in the delivery room and provided a rating of the amount of anxiety that she had experienced during her delivery. Consistent with Masling et al.'s earlier findings, Keinan and Hobfoll found that dependent women were significantly more anxious during delivery when the husband was absent than when he was present. However, nondependent women reported comparable levels of anxiety regardless of whether or not the husband was present during the delivery. Because highly similar results were obtained in samples of American male undergraduates and pregnant Israeli women, these two studies offer strong support for the hypothesis that the presence of others acts as a stress reducer in dependent individuals.

Along different lines, Juni et al. (1979) tested the hypothesis that dependent individuals' affiliative needs would result in increased willingness to touch another person when the experimental situation was constructed to permit interpersonal touching. In this investigation, a mixed-sex sample of undergraduates was divided into dependent and nondependent groups based on ROD scores. Subjects were then asked to participate in a "coaching" task in which they were instructed to guide a blindfolded subject (actually a confederate) through a maze, using whatever techniques (e.g., verbal instructions, physical direction) they chose. Half the subjects were assigned a same-sex confederate and half were assigned an opposite-sex confederate. The number of times that the subject touched the confederate and the total amount of time that the subject spent touching the confederate were recorded covertly by the experimenter.[3]

Juni et al. (1979) found a significant positive correlation between ROD score and the proportion of "coaching" time spent touching the confederate ($r = .39$). Dependent subjects also touched the confederate significantly more frequently than did nondependent subjects. There were no sex differences on either touching measure, nor were there any sex-of-subject by sex of confederate interactions in this experiment. Consistent with Juni et al.'s results, Hollender et al. (1970) found that dependent undergraduate women expressed greater desire than nondependent women for physical contact with their romantic partners. Similarly, Sroufe et al. (1983) found that dependent nursery school children sought physical contact with the teacher more frequently than did nondependent children.[4]

Finally, several studies have tested the hypothesis that dependent persons' affiliative needs would produce increased eye contact with experimenters and interviewers. These studies yielded mixed results, with one experiment (Exline & Messick, 1967) finding greater eye contact with interviewers in dependent than nondependent subjects and three studies finding no relationship between level of dependency and amount of eye contact with interviewers (Burton et al., 1979; Libby & Yanklevich, 1973) or experimenters (Shilkret & Masling, 1981). It seems that there is no strong, consistent relationship between dependency and amount of eye contact with interviewers and experimenters. However, it is difficult to compare these mixed results with other findings regarding the dependency–affiliation link because all investigations of the dependency–eye contact relationship examined subjects' behaviors toward figures of authority, while most other studies in this area assessed subjects' behavior toward peers (Juni et al., 1979; Masling et al., 1982), spouses (Keinan & Hobfoll, 1989), and romantic partners (Hollender et al., 1970; Simpson & Gangestad, 1991).

Although the question of whether dependency predicts the amount of eye contact with an experimenter or interviewer remains unresolved, one subsidiary finding from Exline and Messick's (1967) study deserves mention. Exline and Messick found that dependent subjects were more strongly affected than were nondependent subjects by verbal reinforcement given by the experimenter/interviewer. Specifically, when eye contact was verbally reinforced by the interviewer (who uttered phrases such as "uh-huh," "good," or "right"), dependent subjects showed a significant increase in eye contact. However, nondependent subjects showed no increase in eye contact in response to verbal reinforcement. This result parallels earlier findings by Cairns (1961), Cairns and Lewis (1962), Timmons and Noblin (1963), and Noblin, Timmons, and Kael (1966), each of whom found that dependent persons were more responsive than nondependent persons to similar types of subtle verbal reinforcements provided by a graduate student experimenter in a verbal conditioning paradigm.

Interestingly, Cooperman and Child (1971) found that when a peer (i.e., another undergraduate) rather than a figure of authority (i.e., an older graduate student) served as the experimenter in a verbal conditioning study similar to those conducted by Cairns (1961) and others, no effect of dependency on responsiveness to verbal reinforcement was obtained. As has been found in other areas of dependency research (e.g., in the studies of suggestibility and yielding described earlier), dependent individuals are more responsive to figures of authority than peers in verbal conditioning experiments.

# DEPENDENCY, EVALUATION, AND PERFORMANCE ANXIETY

The results of studies of the dependency–help-seeking relationship raise an interesting question: How will the behavior of dependent individuals be affected when they are forced to work independently and are aware that their performance is being evaluated by a figure of authority? Three experiments have examined the relationship between dependency and performance anxiety in laboratory problem-solving situations (Alam, 1986; Ojha, 1978; Sinha & Pandey, 1972), and three field studies have investigated the relationship between dependency and academic performance (Lao, 1980; Sansanwal, Jarial, & Dandel, 1982; Tesser & Blusiewicz, 1987).

## Dependency and Performance Anxiety

Dependent subjects generally obtain higher scores than do nondependent subjects on self-report and projective measures of performance anxiety. For example, Singh (1981) found that dependent undergraduate subjects (selected according to scores on Sinha's [1968] DP scale) obtained significantly higher scores than did nondependent subjects on a TAT-derived "fear of failure" index.[5] Schlenker and Weigold (1990) similarly found that dependent college students obtained significantly higher scores on Leary's (1983) Fear of Negative Evaluation scale than did nondependent students. Virtually identical findings were obtained by Khan and Sinha (1971). Along the same lines, Devito and Kubis (1983) found that dependent college students (selected according to scores on Navran's [1954] MMPI Dy scale) reported significantly higher levels of test anxiety than did nondependent students. Finally, Goldberg, Segal, Vella, and Shaw (1989) found that dependent psychiatric outpatients (selected according to scores on the MCMI dependency scale [Millon, 1987]) showed greater anxiety regarding evaluation by figures of authority than did nondependent outpatients.

Three laboratory studies of the dependency–performance anxiety relationship produced results consistent with the findings obtained by Singh (1981) and others. In one experiment, Alam (1986) divided 60 undergraduate males into high- and low-dependent groups based on scores on Sinha's (1968) DP scale. He then asked the subjects to memorize a series of briefly presented nonsense syllables in preparation for a recall test. Thirty minutes later, subjects were asked to recall as many of the syllables as possible, in any order. Subjects were tested individually by a male experimenter. Alam found that, as hypothesized, high-DP subjects showed significantly poorer performance on the recall test than did low-DP subjects. He concluded that performance anxiety inhibited the ability of high-DP subjects to recall the previously learned material. However, because performance anxiety was not assessed directly in this study (e.g., by a postexperiment interview or questionnaire), it may be that Alam's results are due to some other factor or combination of factors. For example, it is possible that dependent and nondependent subjects in Alam's experiment recalled the same number of syllables, but that dependent subjects used a higher criterion level for reporting syllables to avoid making any incorrect responses.[6]

Ojha's (1978) findings are consistent with those of Alam (1986), but also suggest that dependent subjects may well utilize higher criterion levels than do nondependent subjects when responding to test items in a typical psychology experiment. In Ojha's investigation, undergraduate male subjects were divided into high- and low-dependent groups using Sinha's (1968) DP scale. Subjects then took part in a choice reaction time (CRT) experiment in which they were asked to indicate as quickly as possible which of two stimulus lights (red or green) was illuminated. Fifteen CRT trials were administered to each subject. Ojha found that high-DP subjects showed significantly slower reaction times than did low-DP subjects. The correlation between DP score and mean CRT in Ojha's study was .32. Sinha and Pandey (1972) similarly obtained a significant positive correlation ($r$ = .53) between undergraduate subjects' DP scores and the amount of time that they took to respond to test items during a laboratory problem-solving task.

Performance anxiety might account for these results, as both Ojha (1978) and Sinha and Pandey (1972) suggested. Alternatively, dependent subjects' slower reaction and response times might reflect a strategy wherein the dependent person is particularly careful and deliberate in responding in order to avoid giving incorrect answers. Clearly, additional work remains to be done to investigate whether findings in this area reflect differences in performance anxiety or differences in response style in dependent and non-dependent subjects. The most that can be said about these results at present is that they are consistent with the hypothesis that dependency is associated with high levels of performance anxiety in laboratory settings when subjects are required to work independently, but that the design of these experiments does not allow alternative interpretations of their findings to be ruled out.

Two other studies are noteworthy in the present context. Juni (1981) found that dependent subjects (selected according to scores on Masling et al.'s [1967] ROD scale) were more likely than nondependent subjects to request feedback regarding their performance in a typical psychology experiment. Juni's result echoes Flanders et al.'s (1961) earlier finding that dependent children ask the teacher for feedback regarding classroom performance more frequently than do nondependent children. Both sets of results are consistent with the hypothesis that dependent subjects have higher levels of performance anxiety than do nondependent subjects, in at least one respect: Obtaining feedback regarding their performance in the classroom or in a psychology experiment may be one way for the dependent individual to reduce the anxiety associated with being evaluated by a figure of authority.

## Dependency and Academic Performance

It is difficult to predict the relationship between dependency and academic performance, because two of the dependency-related traits that are most relevant to academic performance appear to work in opposition to one another. On the one hand, studies by Alam (1986), Ojha (1978), and others suggest that dependency may be associated with performance anxiety, which should hinder academic performance.[7] However, research on the dependency–compliance relationship, described earlier, suggests that dependent individuals are particularly concerned with pleasing figures of authority. This should lead to increased motivation among dependent students to perform well in academic settings in order to please teachers and parents.

Complicating things still further, studies of the relationship between dependency and creativity have yielded conflicting results. Although Holt (1966) and Von Holt, Sengstake, Sanada and Draper (1960) found that dependency was associated with elevated scores on various creativity and concept-formation tests, Blatt, Allison, and Fierstein (1969) used the same projective dependency measure as was used by Holt (1966) and Von Holt et al. (1960) and found a negative relationship between level of dependency and performance on both laboratory and paper-and-pencil problem-solving tasks. In light of (1) the conflicting effects that performance anxiety and compliance are likely to have on academic achievement and (2) the inconsistent findings obtained in studies of the dependency–creativity relationship, it is not surprising that research on dependency and academic performance has also produced mixed results.

In the first study of this issue, Lao (1980) divided a mixed-sex sample of 365 high school students into dependent and nondependent groups based on a self-report measure of interpersonal dependency. She then compared the high school grade-point averages (GPAs) of students in her dependent and nondependent groups, and found that dependent students had significantly lower GPAs overall than did nondependent students. Unfortunately, Lao did not control for academic ability in this study. Thus, it is impossible to ascertain from these results whether dependency actually predicts academic performance or whether the dependent and nondependent students in Lao's sample differed in academic ability.

A similar but better-designed study of this issue was conducted by Tesser and Blusiewicz (1987). They divided a mixed-sex sample of 107 10th graders into dependent and nondependent groups based on scores on a 10-item self-report measure of interpersonal dependency. Academic achievement was assessed by calculating a predicted GPA for each student based on standardized intelligence test scores and then comparing the predicted GPA to the student's actual GPA. A strong relationship between dependency and underachievement was found, with dependent students showing significantly poorer academic performance (i.e., lower GPAs than predicted based on standardized test scores) than nondependent students.

In contrast to the results of Lao (1980) and Tesser and Blusiewicz (1987), Sansanwal et al. (1982) found no relationship between dependency (assessed via scores on Pareek and Rao's [1971] preadolescent dependency scale [PADS]) and academic performance in a sample of 115 female 7th graders. After being prescreened for dependency with the PADS, students participated in an experimental "programmed learning" class. The measure of academic performance in Sansanwal et al.'s (1982) study was the student's score on a post-class achievement test. Sansanwal et al. (1982) found no effect of dependency on achievement test scores in this study. However, because Sansanwal et al.—like Lao—did not control for level of academic ability in this investigation, the implications of their nonsignificant results are difficult to interpret.

Thus, the best-designed study in this area (Tesser & Blusiewicz, 1987) suggests that there is an inverse relationship between dependency and academic performance. Clearly, one would want to see this finding replicated before drawing strong conclusions regarding the dependency–academic performance relationship. However, Tesser and Blusiewicz's results not only are consistent with findings regarding the relationship of dependency to test anxiety and evaluation by figures of authority but further suggest one possible application of dependency research: the early identification of students who might be at risk for scholastic problems. A detailed discussion of potential applications of dependency research is provided in Chapter 10, so I will not elaborate on those issues here. For now, it is sufficient to note that Tesser and Blusiewicz's study is a good example of the ways in which basic theory and research on dependency may be extended into the realm of applied psychology.

## NOTES

1. A related finding reported by Couch and Keniston (1960) should be mentioned in this context. Couch and Keniston examined the relationship between several personality traits and subjects' scores on a self-report measure of acquiescent response set (ARS). They found significant positive correlations between ARS scores and scores on the MMPI Dy scale ($r = .48$), and between ARS scores and scores on a self-report measure of oral dependency ($r = .40$). Insofar as an acquiescent response set reflects a tendency to "[agree] with things authoritative" (Couch & Keniston, 1960, p. 151), these results offer additional support for the dependency–compliance relationship.

2. Although Bernardin and Jessor (1957) used a chi-square statistic to analyze their data while Cairns (1961), Diener (1967), and Sinha and Pandey (1972) used Pearson correlation coefficients to analyze their results, it is possible to convert Bernardin and Jessor's chi-square into a correlation coefficient using the formula provided by Rosenthal (1984). This permits Bernardin and Jessor's findings to be compared directly to those of other researchers. Bernardin and Jessor's chi-square of 10.00 produces an $r$ of .50, somewhat larger than the dependency–help-seeking correlations reported by Diener and Sinha and Pandey, but slightly smaller than the dependency–help-seeking correlation reported by Cairns. Combining the results of these four experiments yields an overall dependency–help-seeking correlation of .44.

3. Although Juni et al.'s (1979) results are consistent with the hypothesis that dependency is associated with affiliative tendencies, a plausible alternative interpretation of these results is worth mentioning. It may be that these findings reflect the dependent individual's concern with doing a "good job" at the experimental task that he or she has been assigned, thereby pleasing the experimenter. Because Juni et al. did not question subjects regarding their feelings and motivations during the experiment, it is impossible to tell whether these findings reflect dependent subjects' affiliative needs, dependent subjects' tendency to comply with the experimenter's expectations, or both of these factors.

4. Interestingly, Fisher and Osofsky (1967) found significant correlations between scores on a self-report measure of oral dependency and estimates of intercourse frequency ($r = .25$), sexual responsiveness ($r = .30$) and orgasm consistency ($r = .25$) in a sample of 42 married women. Although these findings do not address the dependency–affiliation relationship directly, they are nonetheless consistent with the results obtained by Hollender et al. (1970) and others.

5. An interesting footnote to Singh's (1981) study: It was published simultaneously in a different journal, under a different title, and with one coauthor, but with only minor wording changes and no additional data reported (see Singh & Lunyal, 1981).

6. Like Singh's (1981) study, Alam's (1986) study was published simultaneously in a different journal under a different title. In contrast to Singh, who added only one coauthor to his study the second time around, Alam added two coauthors to his study for its "second" publication (see Alam, Khan, & Khan, 1986).

7. In a related vein, two studies examined the relationship between dependency and test anxiety in samples of Indian (Chadha, 1983) and American schoolchildren (Devito & Kubis, 1983). Chadha used Sinha's (1968) DP scale as the measure of dependency in his study, while Devito and Kubis used the MMPI Dy scale (Navran, 1954) as the measure of dependency in their investigation. In both studies, no relationship was found between dependency scores and scores on self-report measures of test anxiety ($r = -.04$ in Chadha's study, and $r = .07$ in Devito & Kubis's study).

# Dependency as a Social Cue

Just as dependency is associated with a number of theoretically-related interpersonal behaviors (e.g., suggestibility, compliance, yielding), dependency can serve as a social cue that influences and directs the behavior of others. Of course, before an individual's dependent behavior can influence others' reactions and responses, the dependent behavior must be noticed and identified by the perceiver as reflecting dependency on the part of the individual exhibiting the behavior. To the extent that dependent behavior is exhibited consistently across different situations and settings, social perceivers are likely to attribute the dependent behavior to internal (i.e., dispositional) causes rather than to external (i.e., situational) variables (Kelley, 1973).

However, research confirms that social perceivers tend to overemphasize dispositional interpretations of others' behavior, even in the face of evidence indicating that situational pressures played a role in determining the behavior in question (the well-known "fundamental attribution error") (see Ross, 1977). Thus, even in situations where an individual's dependent behavior is clearly situationally determined, perceivers will be likely to infer that the behavior actually reflects that individual's underlying dependency needs. Despite social perceivers' tendency to commit the fundamental attribution error in a variety of situations and circumstances, several researchers (e.g., Baker & Reitz, 1978; Harris & Ho, 1984; Horowitz, 1968) have successfully manipulated perceivers' attributions regarding the cause of a target person's dependent behavior and examined the effects of this manipulation on perceivers' responses.

Studies of dependency as a social cue can be divided into three groups. First, researchers have examined the effects of dependency on evaluations by others. These studies have focused primarily on the relationship of dependency to sociometric status (i.e., indices of popularity and peer acceptance). Second, researchers have investigated the effects of the perceived dependency of a target person on others' willingness to offer help and support to that person. Finally, researchers have examined dependency as a factor in child, spousal, and parental abuse.

Before examining the role of dependency as a social cue, it is important to distinguish two general types of dependent behavior that can be exhibited in social settings. First, dependent behavior can stem from genuine feelings of helplessness and dependency. In this situation, dependency is simply an outward manifestation of an individual's internal state (e.g., feelings, motivations). However, dependent behavior can also be exhibited by individuals who do not necessarily *feel* dependent. In other words, dependency can represent a "self-presentation strategy" (Jones & Pittman, 1982) in which an individual chooses to behave in a dependent manner in the hopes that this behavior will elicit support and help from other people.

To date, no researchers have examined differences in the behaviors exhibited by dependent persons and nondependent persons who simply desire to present themselves in a dependent manner. Thus, it is impossible to know whether social perceivers can distinguish these two classes of dependent behavior. In any case, it is clear that individuals who are perceived as being helpless and dependent are treated differently by others than are individuals who are not perceived as being dependent. Keeping in mind that dependent behavior exhibited in social settings may or may not reflect strong underlying dependency needs, I will review the empirical literature examining the dependency–sociometric status, dependency–helping, and dependency–abuse relationships.

## DEPENDENCY AND SOCIOMETRIC STATUS

Six studies have assessed the relationship between dependency and popularity in schoolchildren (Dunnington, 1957; Marshall & McCandless, 1957; McCandless, Bilious, & Bennett, 1961; Miller & Stine, 1951; Moore & Updegraff, 1964; Wiggins & Winder, 1961). These six investigations produced a total of nine dependency–sociometric status comparisons.[1] The results of these studies are summarized in Table 5.1. As this table shows, studies of the dependency–sociometric status relationship have produced highly consistent results: In every study, dependency was associated with a lack of popularity and an absence of social acceptance by peers. Dependency–sociometric status correlations ranged from −.22 (in Miller and Stine's [1951] study) to −.64 (in Dunnington's [1957] investigation), with the mean dependency–sociometric status correlation being −.33. Moreover, comparable dependency–sociometric status correlations were obtained regardless of the type of dependency and sociometric status measures used. Finally, the studies summarized in Table 5.1 indicate that similar depen-

**TABLE 5.1. Studies of Dependency and Sociometric Status**

| Study | Sample | Dependency measure | Sociometric status measure | Dependency–sociometric status correlation |
|---|---|---|---|---|
| Dunnington (1957) | 15 nursery school children | Dependent behavior in structured play situation | Peer ratings | −.64 |
| Marshall & McCandless (1957) | 36 preschool children | Dependent behavior in unstructured classroom situation | Peer rating Teacher ratings Observer ratings | −.34 −.31 −.32 |
| McCandless et al. (1961) | 26 preschool children | Dependent behavior in unstructured classroom situation | Teacher ratings Observer ratings | −.27 −.33 |
| Miller & Stine (1951) | 166 2nd to 7th graders | Projective test (story completion) | Peer ratings | −.22 |
| Moore & Updegraff (1964) | 62 nursery school children | Dependent behavior in unstructured classroom situation | Peer ratings | −.24 |
| Wiggins & Winder (1961) | 710 4th- to 6th-grade boys | Peer and teacher ratings | Peer ratings | −.33 |

*Note.* All studies except that of Wiggins and Winder (1961) used mixed-sex samples. In all studies, higher dependency scores were associated with lower sociometric status ratings.

dency–sociometric status correlations are found in children of various ages (compare, e.g., Marshall and McCandless's [1957] results for preschool children with Wiggins and Winder's [1961] findings for 4th to 6th grade boys).

Gordon and Tegtemeyer (1983) took a different approach to this issue, examining the relationship between dependency and children's perceptions of their own sociometric status. The results of this investigation suggest that dependent children may not be fully aware of their lack of popularity and social acceptance by peers. Subjects in this study were 47 6-year-old children (41 boys and 6 girls), who completed the ROD and a self-report measure of perceived popularity among peers. Gordon and Tegtemeyer found only a small (and nonsignificant) negative correlation ($r = -.13$) between ROD scores and children's estimates of their own popularity.

Interestingly, the results of two investigations suggest that by the time that dependent individuals reach late adolescence, they *are* aware of their lack of popularity and peer acceptance. Mahon (1982) obtained a correlation of .42 between MID dependency scores and self-reports of loneliness in a college student sample, and also found that dependent college students of both sexes reported that they had an inadequate amount of social contact and informal interaction with peers. Similarly, Overholser (1992) found that college student subjects' dependency scores were significantly correlated with self-reports of loneliness and interpersonal isolation (the mean dependency–loneliness correlation for the various subject groups examined in Overholser's study was .22).

The finding that dependency is associated with a lack of popularity and social acceptance by peers is—to say the least—ironic, particularly in light of the fact that much of the dependent person's behavior in social settings is motivated by a desire to be liked and accepted by others. As the studies reviewed in Chapter 4 demonstrated, the dependent person often goes to considerable lengths to minimize interpersonal conflict and to preserve good relationships with other people. In fact, consistent with the findings discussed in Chapter 4, Hartup and Keller (1960) found that dependent schoolchildren exhibited significantly more nurturant, supportive behaviors toward their classmates (e.g., gave more affection, attention, and reassurance) than did nondependent children. Clearly, dependent individuals strive to be accepted by others, but somehow these attempts backfire.

Although no studies have investigated directly the factors underlying the dependency–unpopularity link, some subsidiary findings from Wiggins and Winder's (1961) investigation suggest that immature behaviors exhibited by dependent children may be in part responsible for these children's social isolation and lack of peer acceptance. Wiggins and Winder found that the dependent children in their sample were described by peers as being attention demanding, helpless in a manipulative way, and "babyish." Not surprisingly, these attention-demanding behaviors were most often directed toward teachers rather than toward other children. Beswick and Cox (1958), Blum and Miller (1952), Sears (1963), and Winder and Rau (1962) also found that dependency-related immaturity (particularly immature attention-demanding behavior) was characteristic of the classroom behavior exhibited by dependent boys and girls (see also Birtchnell [1980] for a discussion of some related findings obtained in samples of adult women). Perhaps dependent children's efforts to gain the attention of those individuals who are most likely to be able to offer nurturance, protection, and support (i.e., figures of authority) eventually breed resentment among members of their peer group.

## DEPENDENCY AND HELPING

Paradoxically, although dependency is associated with social rejection by peers, there is strong evidence that dependency also elicits increased helping behavior in others. A number of researchers have assessed the effects of the perceived dependency of a target person on helping behavior (i.e., Baker & Reitz, 1978; Barnes, Ickes, & Kidd, 1979; Berkowitz, 1969; Berkowitz & Connor, 1966; Berkowitz & Daniels, 1963, 1964; Berkowitz, Klanderman, & Harris, 1964; Daniels & Berkowitz, 1963; Gruder, 1974; Gruder & Cook, 1971; Gruder, Romer, & Korth, 1978; Harris & Ho, 1984; Harris & Klingbeil, 1976; Harris & Meyer, 1973; Horowitz, 1968; Jones, 1970; Karasawa, 1991; Midlarsky, 1971; Midlarsky & Midlarsky, 1973; Pandey & Griffitt, 1977; Pomazal & Clore, 1973; Schaps, 1972; Schopler, 1967; Schopler & Bateson, 1965; Schopler & Matthews, 1964; Taylor et al., 1982; Test & Bryan, 1969; Wilke & Lanzetta, 1982; Wolfson, 1981). Typically, these investigations manipulated the degree to which a target person (usually a confederate) was dependent on the subject for assistance, and then assessed the amount of assistance offered to the target person.

Various measures of helping have been used in these investigations, generally producing consistent results. In addition, both laboratory and field studies have found that high levels of target person dependency were associated with increased levels of helping behavior in others. Thus, the dependency–helping relationship appears to generalize across a variety of situations and settings. The various measures and methodologies used in these experiments are too numerous to describe in detail. However, a brief description of several of these measures and experimental manipulations illustrates the kinds of procedures typically used in studies of the dependency–helping relationship.

Baker and Reitz's (1978) investigation was typical of studies in this area. These researchers assessed the degree to which subjects would assist a stranger in completing a telephone call under conditions of high dependency (in which the caller had no more money) or low dependency (in which the caller had the necessary money). Similarly, Wolfson (1981) investigated whether subjects would volunteer to participate in a psychology experiment for no payment or credit under conditions in which the experimenter was highly dependent on the subject's assistance versus conditions wherein the experimenter was less dependent on the subject's help. Using a slightly different approach, Harris and Ho (1984) employed multiple measures of helping in their study, including willingness to help a stranger complete a phone call, to assist an ill (or drunk) stranger on a public street, and to help a student by completing a survey questionnaire. In each situation in Harris and Ho's experiment, level of confederate dependency (i.e., high vs. low) was varied across subjects.

In addition to varying the degree to which the target person was dependent on the subject for help, researchers have examined a number of variables that potentially mediate the dependency–helping relationship. These include the gender of the target person (Gruder & Cook, 1971; Taylor et al., 1982) and that of the subject (Berkowitz et al., 1964; Harris & Ho, 1984); the cost of helping (i.e., high cost vs. low cost) (Gruder, 1974; Schaps, 1972); and the locus of the target person's dependency (i.e., external and beyond the target person's control vs. internal and under the target person's control) (Barnes et al., 1979; Berkowitz, 1969; Gruder et al., 1978). Other experiments have examined the interaction of confederate dependency with the ethnicity of the confederate (Harris & Klingbeil, 1976), or with the degree to which the subject perceived that she had a choice regarding whether to help (i.e., high choice vs. low choice) (Horowitz, 1968).

Berkowitz and his colleagues (e.g., Berkowitz, 1969; Berkowitz & Daniels, 1963, 1964; Berkowitz et al., 1964; Daniels & Berkowitz, 1963) were among the first researchers to investigate empirically the dependency–helping relationship. Most of their studies utilized roughly the same design. Moreover, other researchers examining parameters of the dependency–helping relationship have often used modified versions of the procedures originally devised by Berkowitz and his colleagues. Thus, it is worth describing these experiments in some detail.

In their initial experiment, Berkowitz and Daniels (1963) asked 80 undergraduate males to participate in a study of the characteristics of effective supervisors. The subjects were asked to work at a mundane task (i.e., constructing boxes out of paper and scotch tape) under one of two conditions. Half the subjects were told by their "supervisor" (another male undergraduate) that he was dependent on the subject's performance for a large part of his evaluation as a potential supervisor (the high-dependency condition). The remaining subjects received no information regarding the relationship of subject performance to the evaluation of the supervisor (the low-dependency condition). Berkowitz and Daniels found that as predicted, subjects in the high-dependency condition worked harder (i.e., completed a significantly greater number of boxes) than did subjects in the low-dependency condition.

Later studies of dependency and helping produced results consistent with those of Berkowitz and Daniels (1963), but further indicated that a number of variables mediate the dependency–helping relationship. For example, Schopler and Bateson (1965) found that individuals were more likely to help a dependent person when the cost of helping was low than when it was relatively high. Along different lines, several studies indicated that individuals are more likely to help a dependent person when they believe that the dependency was externally caused and beyond the individual's control (e.g., as in the case of a blind person) than when they believe that the cause of the dependency was within the individual's control (e.g., as in the case of a student who fails to complete his work on time) (see Baker & Reitz, 1978; Barnes et al., 1979; Harris & Ho, 1984; Horowitz, 1968).

Although studies of variables that mediate the dependency–helping relationship have produced fairly consistent results, the same is not true of studies that examine the interaction of subject and target gender on helping. Several experiments (e.g., Schopler, 1967) found that females were more likely than males to help a dependent person, regardless of the gender of the dependent individual (see Berkowitz [1970, 1972] and Krebs [1970] for reviews of early research on the effects of gender and dependency on helping). However, other experiments found that the relationship of gender to helping behavior is more complex than early studies had indicated.

For example, Gruder and Cook (1971) found that dependent female experimenters were more likely to receive help from subjects of both sexes than were nondependent female experimenters, but a parallel relationship was not found for male experimenters. However, Schopler and Bateson (1965) found that males were more likely than females to offer help to a dependent person in both laboratory (Experiments 2 and 3) and field settings (Experiment 1). In an experiment in which volunteering to participate in a psychology experiment for no credit or payment served as the dependent measure of helping, Wolfson (1981) found that both male and female subjects were more likely to help a dependent opposite-sex experimenter than a dependent experimenter of the same sex. To complicate matters still further, Harris and Ho (1984) found that on self-report measures, female subjects reported greater willingness than males to help dependent subjects of both sexes, but in a field experiment wherein actual helping behavior was assessed, males helped subjects of both sexes more often than did females. Finally, Taylor et al. (1982) found no effects of subject or experimenter gender on helping behavior: Subjects of both sexes worked harder to help a dependent experimenter than a nondependent experimenter, regardless of the gender of the experimenter.

Further information regarding the interaction of subject gender, target gender, and target dependency on helping behavior can be obtained by assessing systematically the results obtained under different experimental conditions. Table 5.2 summarizes the results of studies in this area. The 29 studies listed at the beginning of this section yielded a total of 62 separate dependency–helping comparisons. In Table 5.2, these 62 comparisons are grouped by subject and target gender. As this table shows, 41 comparisons (66%) involved male subjects, while 21 comparisons (34%) involved female subjects. Male and female targets were used equally often in these experiments.

Two central conclusions may be drawn from the data in Table 5.2. First, as noted earlier, it is clear that increased target dependency is associated with greater willingness to help on the part of naive subjects. Of the 62 dependency–helping comparisons listed in this table, 37 (60%) produced the predicted results (i.e., significantly greater helping in high-dependent conditions than in low-dependent conditions), while 22 comparisons (35%) yielded no effect of dependency on helping, and only three comparisons (5%) yielded a reverse effect (i.e., significantly greater helping in the low-dependent condition than in the high-dependent condition).

The pattern of results summarized in Table 5.2 also suggests that the dependency–helping relationship is strongest when female subjects and male targets are used. As Table 5.2 shows, 83% of the comparisons in the female–male condition produced the expected results, while the proportion of comparisons that produced the expected results in the female–female, male–male, and male–female conditions were 60%, 60%, and 50%, respectively. It is not clear why this particular pattern of subject and target gender interactions was found in studies of the dependency–helping relationship. These results are inconsistent with Eagly and Crowley's (1986) meta-analytic finding that in studies of helping behavior involving strangers, men typically engage in more helping behavior than do women. The present findings regarding sex differences in the dependency–helping relationship are diametrically opposed to Eagly and Crowley's findings regarding prosocial behavior in general. In fact, these findings are more consistent with recent suggestions by Lerner (1983) and others, who argue that in situa-

TABLE 5.2. Effects of Subject Gender, Target Gender, and Target Dependency on Helping Behavior

| Subject gender | Target gender | Number of comparisons | Dependency–helping relationship | | |
|---|---|---|---|---|---|
| | | | Positive | Absent | Reversed |
| Male | Male | 25 | 15 (60%) | 8 (32%) | 2 (8%) |
| Male | Female | 16 | 8 (50%) | 7 (44%) | 1 (6%) |
| Female | Male | 6 | 5 (83%) | 1 (17%) | 0 (0%) |
| Female | Female | 15 | 9 (60%) | 6 (40%) | 0 (0%) |

*Note.* Positive dependency–helping relationship = significantly more help offered when the target was highly dependent upon the subject than when the target was less dependent on the subject. Negative dependency–helping relationship = significantly less help offered in the high-dependency condition than in the low-dependency condition.

tions involving interpersonal distress, women may be more willing than men to assume an active helping role.

Thus, four general findings have emerged from studies of the dependency–helping relationship. First, researchers have found that dependent individuals typically elicit more help from others than do nondependent individuals in similar situations. Second, studies indicate that the gender of helper and dependent person interact to determine the likelihood of helping behavior, with the greatest amount of helping found when female subjects are confronted with dependent male targets. Third, studies indicate that the likelihood of an individual's helping a dependent person is higher when the cost of helping is low than when the cost of helping is relatively high. Finally, studies suggest that to the extent that an individual's dependency is perceived as externally caused (i.e., beyond the control of the individual), the likelihood that that individual will receive help increases.

Overall, the results of studies of the dependency–helping relationship suggest that behaving in a dependent manner can, in certain situations, be an effective means of obtaining support and assistance from others. In this respect, the dependent person is neither as passive nor as helpless as he or she first appears to be. Nonetheless, while behaving in a dependent manner may be one way of obtaining help and assistance from others, studies of dependency and sociometric status suggest that exhibiting dependent behavior may also entail certain costs (e.g., social isolation and peer rejection). By behaving in a dependent manner, it seems that an individual may be trading long-term success (i.e., popularity and peer acceptance) for short-term gain (i.e., increased help and support from others). This fact alone would indicate that the benefits of exhibiting dependent behavior must be weighed carefully against the costs of appearing to be overly dependent. However, studies of dependency and abuse, which are reviewed in the following section, suggest that behaving in a dependent manner may entail costs that are far more serious than social rejection. These investigations indicate that dependency acts as a social cue that, in certain situations, elicits abusive behavior in others.

## DEPENDENCY AND ABUSIVE BEHAVIOR

Dependency can act as a risk factor for abusive behavior in at least two ways. These two risk factors are described in detail in the following sections, so I will only mention them briefly here. One risk factor reflects the "social cue" aspect of dependency (e.g., dependency exhibited by a nonworking spouse), and the other risk factor is related to the dependency needs of potential abusers. Thus, both "provider" and "providee" dependency may be implicated in child, parental, and spousal abuse.

In this context, numerous researchers have documented the ways in which socioeconomic and emotional dependency increase the likelihood of child (Bennie & Sclare, 1969), spousal (Kalmuss & Straus, 1982), and elder abuse (Pillemer, 1985). The emphasis in these investigations is on the dependency of providees (i.e., children, elderly parents, and nonworking spouses) as a risk factor for abuse. Other investigators have examined the ways in which frustrated dependency needs in caretakers and providers may increase the likelihood that they will engage in abusive behavior directed toward family members (e.g., Kertzman, 1980). The emphasis in these studies is on individual differences in caretaker and provider dependency as a risk factor for abuse.

## Providee Dependency and Caretaker Abuse

The dependency of a child, a nonworking spouse, or an elderly parent on a family member increases the likelihood that the dependent person will become a victim of physical or psychological abuse in several ways. First, supporting and caring for a dependent child, spouse, or parent can be stressful and—on occasion—frustrating. Moreover, the burdens associated with supporting a family member financially and—in the case of children or the elderly—attending to the dependent individual's physical needs can serve as an excuse for engaging in abusive behavior. Abusers may say to themselves, in effect, that they have the right to treat the dependent individual however they please, because the dependent individual survives only as a result of their kindness and goodwill. Anger and frustration can then be displaced onto the dependent family member and rationalized effectively by the abuser. Finally, dependent persons involved in such relationships may believe that they are powerless to change the relationship and yet unable to leave it. In such situations, dependent individuals often believe that they have few options other than remaining in the abusive relationship and tolerating the mistreatment (see Kalmuss & Straus [1982] for an extensive discussion of this issue).

In fact, it appears that the perceived dependency of one family member on another may play as great a role in determining risk for intrafamilial abuse as do more objective indices of dependency. In this context, Kalmuss and Straus (1982) found that both objective dependency and "subjective" (i.e., perceived) dependency were significant factors in risk for spousal abuse. Interestingly, while objective measures of wives' dependency on working husbands (e.g., indices of financial dependency) were strongly correlated with risk for severe abuse in Kalmuss and Straus's study (e.g., serious beatings), subjective dependency indices (e.g., self-reports of emotional dependency) were better predictors of less severe forms of spousal abuse (e.g., slapping, shoving). Overall, 24% of the women in Kalmuss and

Straus's study who reported high levels of objective dependency were victims of some form of abuse, while about 19% of the women who reported high levels of subjective dependency (but not necessarily high levels of objective dependency) were physically abused by their husbands.

## Provider Dependency as a Risk Factor for Abuse

Individual differences in a provider or caretaker's dependency needs can also predict the likelihood that a family member will be subjected to physical or psychological abuse. Numerous writers have speculated that abusive parents and spouses have strong unmet dependency needs (see, e.g., Cochrane, 1965; Gayford, 1975; Laury, 1970; Ponzetti, Cate, & Koval, 1983). Clearly, assuming the caretaker role requires that one allow one's own dependency needs to go unmet. While this may be possible for the individual who does not have a dependent personality orientation, it will be extremely difficult (and frustrating) for the dependent person to relinquish the passive, dependent role in favor of an active, caretaking stance in familial relationships. As Kertzman (1980) noted:

> [T]he continued presence of unsatisfied dependency needs in the parent brings him to focus intensely on his own needs at the expense of his abilities to sympathize with the feelings of others and to form genuine relationships with them . . . the abuser has never had his own [dependency] needs satisfied enough to provide a surplus required for the care of children. (pp. 9–10)

Unfortunately, no studies have examined the relationship of a husband or wife's level of dependency to risk for spousal abuse. However, two studies (Kertzman, 1980; Melnick & Hurley, 1969) examined directly the relationship of parent dependency to risk for child abuse. These two investigations produced highly consistent results. In the first study of this issue, Melnick and Hurley (1969) used the TAT to assess "dependency frustration" in a sample of 10 abusive mothers and in a matched sample of 10 mothers with no history of child abuse or other legal problems. As predicted, the abusive mothers obtained significantly higher scores than did the nonabusing mothers on the TAT dependency frustration index. It is noteworthy that several other personality traits (e.g., need for affiliation, need for dominance, self-reliance) did not distinguish the abusive and nonabusive subjects in Melnick and Hurley's sample.

These results are certainly suggestive, but must be regarded as preliminary, because (1) a relatively small sample of abusive mothers was included in this study and (2) the relationship between dependency and risk for abuse was not examined in fathers. Fortunately, Kertzman (1980) conducted a more extensive investigation of the dependency–abuse relationship, comparing ROD scores in (1) a mixed-sex sample of 40 child-abusing parents currently involved in family court proceedings and (2) a mixed-sex sample of 40 parents who were involved in the family court system for matters unrelated to child abuse or neglect (e.g., to resolve questions regarding custody rights or visitation privileges). Subjects in the two groups were matched on age, race, years of education, socioeconomic status, and number and gender of children. Consistent with the findings of Melnick and Hurley (1969), Kertzman found that abusive parents obtained significantly higher ROD scores than did nonabusing controls. In fact, the ROD scores of abusive parents were nearly twice as great as were the ROD scores of nonabusing control subjects. Moreover, comparable dependency–abuse relationships were found for mothers and fathers in this study, suggesting that Melnick and Hurley's earlier findings generalize to both parents.

It is possible to estimate the magnitude of the dependency–abuse relationship by converting the statistics used by Kertzman (1980) and Melnick and Hurley (1969) into correlation coefficients representing the degree of association between dependency scores and scores on indices of abusive behavior. The main effect of ROD scores on risk for abusive behavior in Kertzman's study converts to an $r$ of .44, suggesting that caretaker dependency might account for as much as 20% of the variance in risk for child abuse. The magnitude of the dependency–abuse relationship reported by Melnick and Hurley was virtually identical to that reported by Kertzman: Melnick and Hurley found a correlation of .45 between TAT dependency frustration scores and risk for child abuse in their subject sample.

Although no studies have examined directly the variables that mediate the dependency–abuse relationship, several investigations have found that dependent individuals show certain traits and behaviors that are linked with risk for child abuse. For example, Agrawal and Rai (1988) found that dependent individuals showed significantly less frustration tolerance than did nondependent individuals in a moderately stressful laboratory problem-solving task. Along different lines, Ederer (1988) found that dependency was associated with low self-esteem, assessed via self-report, while Lorr, Youniss, and Kluth (1992) found that dependency was associated with a lack of openness to new experiences and challenges. Finally, several studies reported that dependent individuals obtain significantly higher scores than do nondependent individuals on various measures of jealousy and insecurity in close relationships (Berscheid & Fei, 1977; Bush, Bush, & Jennings, 1988; Buunk, 1982, 1983; Mathes, Roter, & Joerger, 1982). Thus, in addition to investigating whether Kertzman's (1980) results and Melnick and Hurley's (1969) findings regarding dependency and child abuse generalize to spousal and elder abusers, researchers should now investigate the possibility that low frustration tolerance, low self-esteem, lack of openness to new experiences, and/or high levels of jealousy and insecurity might mediate the dependency–abuse relationship.

## NOTE

1. Winder and Rau (1962, Table 1) also reported data examining the dependency–SES relationship. However, these data were the same as those previously reported by Wiggins and Winder (1961). Thus, only Wiggins and Winder's data are included in Table 5.1.

# CHAPTER 6

# Dependency and Psychopathology

Dependency has been theoretically linked to numerous psychological disorders. These theoretical links are most explicit in the psychoanalytic model (Fisher & Greenberg, 1985; Masling & Schwartz, 1979), but social learning theorists also regard dependency as a risk factor for various psychopathologies (see, e.g., Abramson et al., 1978; Bandura, 1977; Beck, 1967; Dollard & Miller, 1950). Although the dependency–psychopathology relationship has been examined for a wide variety of psychological disorders, research in certain areas has produced inconclusive findings. For example, although there have been several studies assessing the relationship of dependency to risk for schizophrenia (e.g., Aronson, 1953; Devito & Kubis, 1983; DeVos, 1952; Jackson, Rudd, Gazis, & Edwards, 1991b; Rothstein & Cohen, 1958), methodological limitations of these investigations do not allow strong conclusions to be drawn from their results. Similarly, the few studies that assess the relationship of dependency to conversion disorders and hysteria (i.e., Almgren, Nordgren, & Skantze, 1978; Hayward & King, 1990; Mersky & Trimble, 1979) have produced inconsistent, inconclusive findings.

In this chapter, I focus on those disorders that have received substantial attention from dependency researchers. Thus, I will limit my discussion to six categories of psychological disorders. In the following sections I review the empirical literature examining the relationship between dependency and (1) depression; (2) phobias; (3) alcohol abuse and dependence; (4) tobacco dependence; (5) substance use disorders; and (6) obesity and eating disorders.

Before reviewing the empirical literature in these six areas, it is important to place this literature into the proper context by briefly discussing some salient methodological issues. Unfortunately (but predictably), much of the research investigating the dependency–psychopathology relationship has been correlational. This makes it difficult to draw strong conclusions regarding the causal relationship between dependency and the presence of certain disorders. Disentangling the causal relationship between dependency and specific forms of psychopathology is particularly difficult because—as Greenberg and Bornstein (1988b) noted—it is likely that observed dependency–psychopathology relationships reflect at least two factors. First, dependency may place individuals at risk for certain disorders. Second, the onset of certain disorders (e.g., depression, alcoholism) may produce an increase in dependent feelings and behaviors. Thus, in reviewing the dependency–psychopathology literature, it is important to distinguish correlational studies that examine the *association* of dependency with various forms of psychopathology from experimental and prospective studies that assess the *causal relationship* between dependency and various types of psychopathology.

With this in mind, it is clear that for any given disorder there are four possible dependency–psychopathology relationships. First, dependency may be a risk factor for a particular disorder, predicting symptom onset and/or the severity of symptoms. Second, increases in dependent feelings, thoughts, and behaviors may follow the onset of a disorder. Third, studies might confirm that there is a correlation between level of dependency and level of psychopathology but provide no information regarding causal relationships between these variables. Finally, dependency may be unrelated to a particular form of psychopathology. A review of the empirical literature reveals that the dependency–psychopathology relationship differs for different disorders.

## DEPENDENCY AND DEPRESSION

There have been dozens of correlational studies assessing the relationship between level of dependency and the presence (or severity) of depression (e.g., Andrews & Brown, 1988; Blatt, D'Afflitti, & Quinlan, 1976; Blatt et al., 1982; Brewin & Furnham, 1987; Brown & Silberschatz, 1989; Chevron et al., 1978; Hirschfeld et al., 1977; Hirschfeld, Klerman, Clayton, & Keller, 1983; Hirschfeld, Klerman, Clayton, Keller, & Andreason, 1984; Hirschfeld et al., 1989; Hokanson & Butler, 1992; Klein, 1989; Klein, Harding, Taylor, & Dickstein, 1988; Navran, 1954; O'Neill & Bornstein, 1990, 1991; Overholser, 1991; Pilkonis & Frank, 1988; Pilowski, 1979; Pilowski & Katsikitis, 1983; Robins, 1990; Robins & Block, 1988; Robins, Block, & Peselow, 1989; Rossman, 1984; Smith, O'Keeffe, & Jenkins, 1988; Talbot, Duberstein, & Scott, 1991; Welkowitz et al., 1985; Whiffen & Sasseville, 1991; Zuroff, Igreja, & Mongrain, 1990; Zuroff & Mongrain, 1987). The vast majority of these investigations found a significant positive relationship between level of dependency and level of depression.[1]

The dependency–depression relationship has been obtained with a variety of depression scales (e.g., the Beck Depression Inventory [BDI] [Beck, 1967], the MMPI Dy scale, the Zung Depression Scale [ZDS] [Zung, 1965]), and with a variety of dependency measures (e.g., the ROD, the MID, the DEQ dependency scale). In addition, a few investigations have used indirect, behavioral measures of depression (e.g., Juni, Nelson, & Brannon, 1986). These studies generally produced results consistent with those obtained in studies of the dependency–depression relationship that used more traditional interview and self-report depression measures.

It also appears that the dependency–depression relationship is consistent across different subject groups. Specifically, the dependency–depression relationship is found in nonclinical subjects (Robins, 1990; Zuroff & Mongrain, 1987), in members of clinical (i.e., psychiatric inpatient and outpatient) populations (Hirschfeld et al., 1977, 1983; O'Neill & Bornstein, 1991), and in samples of hospitalized medical patients (Brown & Rawlinson, 1975). Moreover, comparable dependency–depression relationships are found in children (Wiggins & Winder, 1961) and adults (Chevron et al., 1978). Finally, the dependency–depression relationship is found in both women and men. However, the magnitude of the dependency–depression relationship is somewhat stronger in men than in women (Blatt et al., 1976, 1982; Chevron et al., 1978; Klein, 1989; O'Neill & Bornstein, 1991).

Information regarding the overall magnitude of the dependency–depression relationship was provided by Nietzel and Harris (1990), who conducted a meta-analysis of studies assessing the co-occurrence of dependency and depression in various subject groups. Mean dependency–depression score correlations in Nietzel and Harris's study sample ranged from .19 (for studies using the ZDS [Zung, 1965] as a measure of depression) to .33 (for studies using the BDI [Beck, 1967] and Hopkins Symptom Checklist [SCL-90] [Derogatis, Lipman, & Covi, 1973]). A few investigations have obtained somewhat higher dependency–depression correlations than those reported by Nietzel and Harris. For example, Brown and Silberschatz (1989) obtained a correlation of .53 between DEQ dependency scores and BDI scores in members of a psychiatric outpatient sample, while O'Neill and Bornstein (1991) found a correlation of .50 between ROD scores and MMPI Dy scores in a sample of male psychiatric inpatients, and Wiggins and Winder (1961) reported a correlation of .62 between peer ratings of dependency and level of depression in a sample of elementary school students. Although there is some variability in the magnitude of the dependency–depression link obtained in different studies, overall the association between dependency and depression is best described as being in the small to moderate range (Rosenthal, 1984). Dependency scores typically account for 10–20% of the variance in depression scores.

The modest correlation between dependency and depression is not surprising. Clearly, dependency is only one of many factors that may play a role in the etiology and dynamics of this disorder. Furthermore, certain forms of depression (e.g., depression characterized by passivity, anergia, and helplessness) should be more strongly associated with dependency than are other forms of the disorder (e.g., agitated depression). Unfortunately, studies in this area typically have not distinguished subtypes of depression before assessing the dependency–depression relationship (cf. Birtchnell & Kennard, 1983; Blatt et al., 1976; Pilowski & Katsikitis, 1983; Robins et al., 1989; Rossman, 1984; Zuroff et al., 1990). Thus, the degree of association between dependency and different forms of depression remains largely unexplored.

There are three plausible interpretations of the observed dependency–depression link. First, some researchers have suggested that dependency somehow predisposes individuals to depression (see O'Neill & Bornstein [1991] for a summary of this view). Second, some researchers have argued that dependency is a product of depression, following rather than preceding the onset of depressive symptomatology (Akiskal, Hirschfeld, & Yerevanian, 1983). Finally, some researchers suggest that depression and dependency are both products of some underlying variable (e.g., a dysfunctional attributional style) (see Abramson et al., 1978).

Although research has demonstrated that dependency levels of formerly depressed individuals remain somewhat elevated even after depressive symptomatology is no longer present (see Frank, Kupfer, Jacob, & Jarrett, 1987; Hirschfeld et al., 1983, 1984; Overholser, 1990; Reich, Noyes, Hirschfeld, Coryell, & O'Gorman, 1987; Reich & Troughton, 1988; Wittenborn & Maurer, 1977), experimental and quasi-experimental studies also indicate that dependency levels and depression levels covary in normal and clinical subjects. Specifically, research has demonstrated that changes in level of depression are associated with changes in dependent thoughts, feelings, and behaviors (Hirschfeld et al., 1983; Hirschfeld, Klerman, Andreason, Clayton, & Keller, 1986; Joffe & Regan, 1988; Klein et al., 1988; Rossman, 1988). Conversely, manipulation of underlying dependency needs produces changes in subjects' depression levels (Zuroff & Mongrain, 1987).

Klein et al. (1988) conducted one of the most extensive and well-designed studies of this issue. Using a longitudinal approach, Klein et al. examined the dependency–depression relationship in a sample of 78 female subjects, 63 of whom were undergoing outpatient treatment for depression, and 15 of whom had no lifetime history of psychopathology or psychological treatment. DEQ dependency scores and clinical depression ratings were collected from subjects at the start of the study, and again 6 months later. Klein et al. found that—as predicted—depressed subjects showed significantly higher dependency scores than did control subjects. However, depressed subjects who showed a remission of depressive symptoms at 6-month follow-up also showed a significant decrease in DEQ dependency scores from Time 1 to Time 2. In contrast, depressed subjects who showed little or no change in depression level from Time 1 to Time 2 also showed no change in dependency scores during the course of the study.

Virtually identical findings were obtained by Hirschfeld et al. (1983). They found significant decreases in both MID scores (Hirschfeld et al., 1977) and LK oral dependency scores (Lazare et al., 1966, 1970) in a mixed-sex sample of depressed inpatients who showed a remission of depressive symptoms at 1-year follow-up. However, consistent with the findings of Klein et al. (1988), Hirschfeld et al. (1983) found no significant changes in MID or LK scores in those depressed patients who showed no improvement during the course of the study. Hirschfeld et al. (1986) subsequently found similar but weaker results in a mixed-sex sample of depressed psychiatric inpatients. Paralleling the findings of Klein et al. (1988) and Hirschfeld et al. (1983, 1986), Stein and Sanfilipo (1985) found that changes in depression level predicted changes in overt dependent behaviors in a mixed-sex sample of nonclinical subjects. Rossman (1988) similarly found that changes in depression level were associated with changes in dependency scores in a sample of Austrian army recruits.

Although the majority of investigations in this area found that decreases in depressive symptoms were associated with decreases in dependency scores, at least one study has produced conflicting results regarding this issue. Stankovic, Libb, Freeman, and Roseman (1992) used the MCMI (Millon, 1987) to assess pre- and posttreatment dependency levels in members of a mixed-sex sample of depressed outpatients. In contrast to other studies in this area, Stankovic et al. found no significant change in subjects' MCMI dependency scores from pre- to posttreatment.

It is impossible to tell whether the contrasting results obtained by Stankovic et al. (1992) are due to differences in the way that dependency was assessed in this study relative to other investigations in this area or whether these results reflect differences in the characteristics of the subjects examined in this study relative to those examined in other studies. At any rate, it is clear that the majority of studies conducted to date have found that dependency and depression scores covary in psychiatric inpatients, outpatients, and nonclinical subjects. Although Stankovic et al.'s results are inconsistent with other findings in this area, it is important to note that even in this investigation, a small (albeit nonsignificant) positive correlation ($r = .10$) was obtained between changes in subjects' depression scores and changes in their dependency scores from pre- to posttreatment.

While there have been a number of studies examining the covariation of depression and dependency scores in various subject groups, only one investigation has manipulated subjects' underlying dependency needs directly and examined the impact of this manipulation on subjects' depression levels. Zuroff and Mongrain (1987) selected dependent and nondependent female undergraduates according to scores on the DEQ dependency scale. Subjects then listened to one of two audiotaped interpersonal interactions. In one interaction, which was intended to be particularly upsetting to the dependent subjects, a woman was rejected by her boyfriend (the "rejection" audiotape). In the other interaction, which was designed to be upsetting to self-critical rather than dependent subjects, a woman's graduate school application was turned down (the "failure" audiotape). Following exposure to the audiotapes, subjects completed several measures of state (i.e., transient) depression. Zuroff and Mongrain found that dependent subjects showed significantly higher depression levels following exposure to the "rejection" audiotape than following exposure to the "failure" audiotape. Furthermore, dependent subjects showed significantly higher depression levels than did nondependent subjects following exposure to the "rejection" audiotape. As predicted, dependent subjects did not show increased depression relative to nondependent subjects following exposure to the "failure" audiotape.

Zuroff and Mongrain's (1987) results suggest that only certain types of stressful events (e.g., those related to interpersonal rejection) produce increased depression in dependent persons. Apparently, dependency acts as a diathesis that—when coupled with events in the environment that activate dependent feelings—predicts changes in depressive symptomatology. In this context, several experiments have examined the interaction of dependency and stressful life events as predictors of depression (Hammen, Ellicott, & Gitlin, 1989a; Hammen, Ellicott, Gitlin, & Jamison, 1989b; Hammen, Marks, Mayol, & DeMayo, 1985; Overholser, 1992; Robins, 1990; Robins & Block, 1988; Smith et al., 1988).

In the first study of this issue, Hammen et al. (1985) divided a mixed-sex sample of college students into dependent and nondependent groups based on DEQ dependency scores. Four months later, subjects reported the number of negative interpersonal events (e.g., rejection by a friend) and negative achievement-related events (e.g., failure on a test) that they had experienced since the first session. Level of depression at follow-up was assessed via the BDI. Hammen et al. (1985) found that dependent subjects reported elevated levels of depression at follow-up only when they had experienced high levels of interpersonal stressors. There was no relationship between depression scores and level of stressful achievement-related events in dependent subjects. Furthermore, nondependent subjects who experienced high levels of negative interpersonal events did not show elevated levels of depression at follow-up. These findings not only support the hypothesis that dependency interacts with stressful life events to predict the onset of depressive symptoms, but further suggest that—consistent with the findings of Zuroff and Mongrain (1987)—only those negative life events that are specifically related to dependent feelings and dependency needs produce increased depression in dependent individuals.

When Hammen et al. (1989a, 1989b) conducted modified replications of this study using psychiatric inpatients and outpatients instead of normal subjects, they obtained very similar results. Again, high levels of interpersonal stressors predicted increases in depressive symptomatology in dependent patients only. Other kinds of stressors did not influence depressive symptoms in Hammen et al.'s (1989a, 1989b) dependent patients, and interpersonal stressors did not predict changes in depression levels in nondependent patients. Robins (1990) obtained similar results in mixed-sex samples of psychiatric patients (Experiment 1) and undergraduates (Experiment 2). Overholser (1992) also found that dependency and stressful life events (in this case, experiences of interpersonal loss) combined to predict depression levels in a mixed-sex sample of undergraduate subjects.

Robins and Block (1988) and Smith et al. (1988) also obtained similar results in mixed-sex undergraduate samples, although in both of these studies a variety of stressful life events—not only those events related to interpersonal stress—interacted with preexisting dependency levels to predict the onset of depressive symptomatology. Thus, while the majority of studies in this area indicate that dependency and negative interpersonal events interact to predict level of depression in both clinical and nonclinical subjects, the results of Robins and Block's (1988) and Smith et al.'s (1988) investigations suggest that other types of stressful life events may also lead to increased depression in dependent individuals. It may be that some of the achievement-related stressful life events assessed in the Robins and Block and Smith et al. studies actually had an adverse impact on subjects' interpersonal relationships, thereby increasing depression levels in dependent subjects (e.g., for some subjects, problems at work might have had a negative effect on relationships at home). However, this possibility has not been addressed.

One final issue regarding the dependency–life stress–depression relationship warrants mention. Although a number of investigations have demonstrated that dependency and stressful interpersonal events interact to predict depression levels in various subject groups, some recent findings reported by Hammen (1991) indicate that depression may also play a role in the generation of interpersonal stress. Using a prospective design, Hammen assessed the number, type, and severity of stressful life events in samples of depressed women ($n = 14$), women with bipolar disorder ($n = 11$), women with chronic medical illnesses ($n = 13$), and women with no medical or psychiatric disorders ($n = 22$). The results of this investigation were clear: During the 1-year course of the study, depressed women reported significantly more stressful interpersonal events than did women in any other group, and they also reported experiencing significantly more dependency-related stressors than did women in any other group. Not only do stressful interpersonal events contribute to the onset of depression in dependent individuals, but depression may also contribute to the onset of stressful interpersonal events, as well as predicting the occurrence of dependency-related life events.

Three recent studies (Bornstein, Greenberg, Leone, & Galley, 1990; Levit, 1991; Mongrain & Zuroff, 1989) suggest a possible cognitive link in the dependency–life events–depression relationship. In the first of these studies, Mongrain and Zuroff assessed level of dependency in a mixed-sex undergraduate sample, using the DEQ dependency scale. Subjects then completed the Dysfunctional Attitudes Scale (DAS) (Weissman & Beck, 1978), which assesses (among other things) maladaptive dependency-related thought patterns (see Mongrain & Zuroff [1989] for a complete list of dependency-related DAS items). Finally, subjects estimated the level of stress that they believed they would experience in response to two types of negative life events: interpersonal and achievement related. Dependency scores and DAS scores interacted to predict subjects' ratings of stressful interpersonal life events: Dependent subjects with high DAS scores perceived negative interpersonal life events as more stressful than did subjects in any other group. However, dependency and DAS scores were unrelated to perceptions of negative achievement-related events.

Bornstein et al.'s (1990) study of defense-mechanism correlates of dependency suggests another possible link in the dependency–life stress–depression relationship. Bornstein et al. (1990) assessed level of dependency in two mixed-sex samples of undergraduate subjects, using Masling et al.'s (1967) ROD scale to measure dependency in one sample and the LK oral dependency scale (Lazare et al., 1966, 1970) to measure dependency in the other sample. Subjects in both samples also completed the Defense Mechanisms Inventory (DMI) (Gleser & Ihilevich, 1969), which asks subjects to report their most and least likely responses to various interpersonal conflicts. Subjects' DMI responses are then used to derive scores on various indices of defensive style (see Ihilevich & Gleser [1986] and Gleser & Ihilevich [1969] for detailed discussions of DMI scoring and interpretation).

Bornstein et al. (1990) found significant negative correlations between dependency score and DMI "turning against object" (TAO) score in both subject samples. In addition, in both samples dependency score was inversely related to score on the DMI index of "outward-directed aggression" (AGG). Finally, in both samples dependency score was positively correlated with DMI "turning against self" (TAS) score (an index of inward-directed anger and frustration). Bornstein et al.'s (1990) results indicate that dependent individuals respond to interpersonal conflict by directing anger and aggression inward rather than expressing their anger directly. Virtually identical findings were subsequently obtained by Levit (1991) in a mixed-sex sample of high school students.[2]

Thus, studies by Mongrain and Zuroff (1989), Bornstein et al. (1990), and Levit (1991) suggest that the dependency–life stress–depression relationship may be mediated by dysfunctional beliefs and attitudes regarding interpersonal stressors and by a defensive style characterized by inward-directed (rather than openly expressed) anger, aggression, and frustration. Clearly, these results must be regarded as preliminary, and further research is needed to explore more fully the relationship of dependency, stressful life events, and depression. However, based on the available data, it seems clear that (1) dependency is associated with elevated levels of depression; (2) changes in depression are associated with parallel changes in dependent feelings and behaviors (and vice versa); (3) dependency interacts with dependency-related stressful life events (e.g., interpersonal rejection) to predict changes in depression level; and (4) dysfunctional attitudes and/or a maladaptive defensive style may mediate the dependency–life stress–depression relationship.

## DEPENDENCY AND PHOBIAS

Numerous psychoanalytic writers have hypothesized that dependency underlies the development of phobic disorders (see, e.g., Fenichel, 1945; Ruddick, 1961). Kleiner and Marshall (1985) summarized nicely the classical psychoanalytic view of phobias, noting that the phobic individual "is thought to regress emotionally to infantile dependence, and their partner in a relationship is said to substitute for the mother and allay this anxiety and dependency" (p. 582). Other writers have interpreted the dependency–phobias link within a social learning framework, suggesting that insofar as traditional sex-role socialization practices encourage and reinforce dependent traits and behaviors in women, these socialization practices may also play a role in the development of phobias (Parker, 1983; Symonds, 1971). Still other researchers have adopted a more behavioral view, hypothesizing that phobia-related dependency—like phobias themselves—may be acquired via conditioning (i.e., through reinforcement of passive, dependent behaviors within the context of the parental or marital relationship) (see Goldstein, 1970; Goldstein & Chambless, 1978).

In light of the fact that several theoretical frameworks hypothesize that a connection should exist between dependency and phobic behavior, it is not surprising that there have been a number of empirical studies of the dependency–phobia relationship. Several studies have examined the relationship of dependency to school phobia, and several studies have investigated the dependency–agoraphobia link. Research in these two areas will be considered separately.

## School Phobia

In a series of investigations conducted during the late 1960s and early 1970s, Berg and his colleagues found that dependency was associated with elevated rates of school phobia in elementary and junior high school students (Berg, 1974; Berg & McGuire, 1974; Berg, McGuire, & Whelan, 1973; Berg, Nichols, & Pritchard, 1969). Comparable dependency–school phobia relationships were obtained in boys and girls in these studies. Furthermore, Berg et al. (1969) found that "chronic" school phobics (i.e., those children who showed clinically significant school phobia for at least 3 consecutive years) obtained significantly higher dependency scores than did "acute" school phobics. Berg and McGuire (1974) subsequently found that mothers of school-phobic children reported more overprotective attitudes and behaviors than did mothers of nonphobic children. Specifically, mothers of school-phobic children reported (1) desiring more contact with their children; (2) desiring greater expressions of affection from their children; and (3) discouraging independent, autonomous behavior in their children in several areas (e.g., when completing school assignments, when traveling outside the home).

Because all studies of the dependency–school phobia relationship conducted to date have been correlational, it is impossible to know whether dependency precedes or follows the onset of school-phobic behavior. However, Berg and McGuire's (1974) findings regarding maternal overprotectiveness in school-phobic children suggest one possible causal link in the dependency–school phobia relationship. Studies by Baumrind (1967, 1971) and others (e.g., Levy, 1943; Parker, 1983) suggest that maternal overprotectiveness instills in a child the belief that he or she cannot function independently and without assistance from others. Thus, maternal overprotectiveness may simultaneously (1) reinforce school-phobic behaviors and (2) encourage the child to view him- or herself as dependent on others for nurturance, help, and support. In this respect, Berg and McGuire's findings regarding school phobias in children parallel the results of studies that suggest that parental overprotectiveness and reinforcement of passive dependency are associated with high levels of dependency in children, adolescents, and adults (e.g., Fu et al., 1986; Kagan & Moss, 1960; Parker & Lipscombe, 1980).

One final issue regarding the dependency–school phobia relationship warrants mention. Because school phobia represents in part a form of exaggerated attachment behavior (i.e., insecure attachment coupled with pronounced separation anxiety), it is important to examine closely the dependency measure used by Berg and his colleagues to rule out the possibility that this measure taps attachment behaviors in addition to (or in lieu of) dependent behaviors. Berg et al.'s (1969) dependency questionnaire consists of a series of likert-type ratings of the child's behavior; ratings are made by the child's primary caretaker. Scrutiny of the items that compose this questionnaire confirms that the measure taps dependency and is relatively free from attachment-related confounds. For example, typical items on Berg et al.'s questionnaire include: "Did he/she talk things over with you and ask your help with what was going on with his/her friends?" and "Did you put out clothes for him/her that it would have been possible for him/her to get himself/herself?" Thus, the findings of Berg and his colleagues genuinely support the hypothesis that dependency is associated with school phobia and do not simply represent positive correlations between two different indices of attachment behavior.

## Agoraphobia

Findings regarding the relationship of dependency to agoraphobia are generally consistent with findings regarding the dependency–school phobia link. Studies in this area have demonstrated that agoraphobic psychiatric patients obtain significantly higher scores than do nonphobic control patients on a variety of dependency measures (Reich, Noyes, & Troughton, 1987; Shafar, 1970; Torgerson, 1979; cf. Sciuto et al., 1991). However, the specificity of the dependency–agoraphobia relationship in adults remains uncertain: While Shafar found that agoraphobic outpatients obtained significantly higher dependency scores (assessed via clinicians' ratings and interviews with family members) than did patients with other types of phobias, Torgerson found that patients with other phobic disorders (e.g., simple phobias) obtained LK oral dependency scores comparable to those of agoraphobic patients. Similarly, when Alnaes and Torgerson (1988b) assessed DPD symptomatology via structured clinical interview in a mixed-sex sample of 289 psychiatric outpatients, high levels of DPD symptomatology were found in agoraphobic patients, in patients with social phobias, and in patients with simple phobias. Furthermore, Alnaes and Torgerson found that levels of DPD symptoms were actually higher in patients with social phobias than in patients with agoraphobia or simple phobias (see also Stewart, Knize, & Pihl [1992] for related findings regarding this issue).

Only one study compared dependency scores in phobic patients versus patients with other types of anxiety disorders. Reich et al. (1987) divided a mixed-sex sample of 88 psychiatric outpatients with DSM-III-R anxiety disorders into three groups: (1) patients with no agoraphobic features ($n =$ 29); (2) patients with moderate/limited agoraphobia ($n = 23$); and (3) patients with severe agoraphobia ($n = 36$). Three measures of dependency were administered to each patient: the MCMI dependency scale (Millon, 1987); the Personality Diagnostic Questionnaire-Revised (PDQ-R) (Hyler et al., 1988); and a structured clinical interview designed to obtain information related to DPD symptoms. Reich et al. (1987) found that agoraphobic patients obtained significantly higher dependency scores on all three measures than did nonagoraphobic anxiety disorder patients or patients with moderate/limited agoraphobia. Moreover, although women showed higher overall rates of agoraphobia than men in Reich et al.'s sample, comparable dependency–agoraphobia relationships were found in men and women.

Mavissakalian and Hamann's (1986) investigation provides further evidence regarding the specificity of the dependency–agoraphobia link, although a somewhat different strategy was used in this investigation than was used in Reich et al.'s (1987) study. Mavissakalian and Hamann compared the prevalence of DPD symptoms and diagnoses with the prevalence of other personality disorder symptoms and diagnoses in a sample of 60 agoraphobic psychiatric patients. Personality disorder symptoms were assessed via the PDQ-R (Hyler et al., 1988). Mavissakalian and Hamann found that—as predicted—dependent, avoidant, and histrionic personality disorder symptoms were most prevalent in their agoraphobic subjects. Fifteen percent of the agoraphobic subjects in this sample scored above the PDQ-R clinical threshold for DPD, while 17% of the subjects scored above the clinical threshold for avoidant personality disorder and 12% of the subjects scored above the clinical threshold for histrionic personality disorder. No more than 3% of the subjects in Mavissakalian and Hamann's sample scored above the clinical threshold score for any other personality disorder.

The studies discussed thus far suggest that dependency is associated with agoraphobia. In addition, it appears that other types of phobias may also be associated with elevated levels of dependency. However, the investigations reviewed thus far have not addressed the causal relationship between dependency and phobias. Only two studies (Buglass, Clarke, Henderson, Kreitman, & Presley, 1977; Mavissakalian & Hamann, 1987) examined this issue directly. These investigations used very different procedures and measures of dependency and produced somewhat different results.

In the first study of this issue, Buglass et al. (1977) assessed the premorbid adjustment of 30 agoraphobic women and 30 matched control subjects with no history of psychiatric disorders. Premorbid traits and behaviors were assessed via a structured clinical interview administered to the patients and controls. Interview questions focused on the subject's early relationship with her mother and on the numbers and types of conformity behaviors exhibited in school. Buglass et al. (1977) found no differences between agoraphobics and matched controls in self-reports of premorbid dependency. This suggests that increases in dependency may follow, rather than precede, the onset of agoraphobic symptoms. However, because retrospective reports of dependency were used in this investigation, it is possible that Buglass et al.'s (1977) negative findings were due, in whole or in part, to interviewee bias and selective reporting of dependency-related childhood behaviors. Furthermore, it appears that the interview questions used by Buglass et al. (1977) assessed individual differences in attachment behaviors as well as differences in dependency, making it even more difficult to interpret the results of their study with respect to the dependency–agoraphobia relationship.

Mavissakalian and Hamann (1987) took a different approach to this issue, comparing PDQ-R Dependency scores (Hyler et al., 1988) collected from 33 agoraphobic patients (1) before the patients underwent treatment for their phobic disorders and (2) following 16 weeks of combined pharmacological and behavioral treatment. Mavissakalian and Hamann found a 25% reduction in dependency scores from pre- to posttreatment. However, even at posttreatment, dependency scores remained significantly elevated and were higher than all other PDQ-R scores except those of avoidant personality disorder. Interestingly, when Mavissakalian and Hamann classified their agoraphobic subjects into "responders" and "nonresponders" based on the amount of agoraphobia symptom reduction that occurred during treatment, they found that the nonresponders had significantly higher pretreatment dependency scores than did the responders. Apparently, high levels of dependency are associated with unfavorable treatment outcome in agoraphobics (see Frank et al. [1987] for a discussion of similar findings in a sample of depressed patients).

Thus, studies conducted to date confirm that dependency is associated with elevated levels of phobic symptomatology, but the limitations of this relationship remain open to question. In particular, the specificity of the dependency–school phobia and dependency–agoraphobia links warrant further study. Nonetheless, the finding that dependency is associated with school phobia in children and with agoraphobia in adults is consistent with Keinan and Hobfoll's (1989) finding (discussed in detail in Chapter 4) that the presence of significant others acts as a stress reducer in dependent individuals. Both school phobia and agoraphobia are characterized by a strong desire to remain in the relative safety of the home, around those individuals with whom the phobic person feels secure. Thus, results in this area offer additional support for the hypothesis that dependent individuals seek the support and comfort of others when they feel anxious or threatened.

## DEPENDENCY AND ALCOHOLISM

Several lines of evidence suggest that dependency might be associated with alcohol abuse and dependence. Classical psychoanalytic theory postulates a dependency–alcoholism link in that dependent individuals are hypothesized to rely on "oral" activities (e.g., drinking, eating, smoking) to cope with anxiety (Bertrand & Masling, 1969). Consistent with this hypothesis, dependent and alcoholic individuals obtain similar scores on a variety of personality measures (e.g., depression, field dependence, various defense mechanism scales) (see Ihilevich & Gleser, 1986; O'Neill et al., 1984; Taccoen & Ansoms, 1980). Furthermore, dependent individuals obtain low scores on measures of ego strength (Nacev, 1980), self-esteem (Ederer, 1988; Overholser, 1992), and perceived self-efficacy (Bornstein et al., 1988a), all of which are associated with increased risk for alcohol abuse and dependence (Vaillant, 1983). Finally, anthropological evidence indirectly supports the hypothesized dependency–alcoholism link: Bacon, Barry, and Child's (1965) cross-cultural data indicate that alcoholism rates in different cultures show a strong inverse relationship with the degree to which caretakers affirm and gratify dependency needs during infancy and early childhood.

Numerous correlational studies confirm that there is an association between alcoholism and dependency (Bertrand & Masling, 1969; Button, 1956; Conley, 1980; Craig, Verinis, & Wexler, 1985; Lawlis & Rubin, 1971; Lemert, 1962; Poldrugo & Forti, 1988; Spolter, Tokar, & Gocka, 1978; Taccoen & Ansoms, 1980; Tognazzo, 1970; Weiss & Masling, 1970; Wiener, 1956; Wolowitz & Barker, 1968; cf. Blane & Chafetz, 1971; Evans, 1984; McCord et al., 1962). In the majority of these investigations, alcoholic subjects obtain significantly higher dependency scores than do nonalcoholic subjects (i.e., abstainers or social drinkers), even when potential confounding variables (e.g., overall level of psychopathology) are controlled for statistically. Of course, these correlational studies do not address the question of whether dependency actually predisposes individuals to alcohol abuse or dependence. Dependency might well predict risk for alcoholism, but an equally plausible interpretation of these data is that alcoholism somehow causes an increase in dependent feelings, thoughts, and behaviors.

Longitudinal studies of the dependency–alcoholism relationship clearly support the latter hypothesis. Jones (1968, 1971), Kammeier, Hoffman, and Loper (1973), and Vaillant (1980) conducted prospective studies of the dependency–alcoholism relationship and obtained highly consistent results. In these investigations, premorbid dependency levels did not predict subsequent risk for alcoholism. However, Vaillant found that a variety of dependency-related traits (i.e., dependent thoughts, feelings and behaviors, passivity, pessimism, self-doubt) showed a significant increase following the onset of alcoholism in his sample of male subjects who were assessed periodically on a variety of personality and psychopathology measures between the ages of 20 and 50.

Although the available data suggest that dependency results from (rather than predisposing individuals to) alcohol abuse or dependence, the results of one study (Spolter et al., 1978) suggest that dependency might predict recidivism following alcoholism treatment. Spolter et al. (1978) utilized the EPPS succorance scale as a measure of dependency, obtaining EPPS scores from 104 male Veterans Administration (VA) patients undergoing inpatient treatment for alcohol addiction. Spolter et al. (1978) then compared the dependency scores of patients who returned for additional inpatient treatment within the first 6 months after discharge ($n$ = 73) with the dependency scores of patients who did not seek further treatment for alcohol problems during the 6-month postdischarge period ($n$ = 31). Dependency predicted alcoholic recidivism in this study: As predicted, the patients who returned for additional treatment had significantly higher dependency scores than the patients who did not seek further treatment.

It is possible, as Spolter et al. (1978) suggested, that dependency is a factor in alcoholic recidivism. However, it is also possible that the dependent and nondependent patients in Spolter et al.'s study actually showed comparable relapse rates, but that dependent patients were more willing than nondependent patients to seek further treatment following relapse. Shilkret and Masling's (1981) finding (described in Chapter 4) that dependent individuals show elevated rates of help-seeking behaviors supports the latter interpretation of Spolter et al.'s (1978) results.

Recently, several investigators have attempted to identify separate dependent subtypes among groups of alcoholic patients (Corbisiero & Reznikoff, 1991; McMahon, Davidson, Gersh, & Flynn, 1991; Poldrugo & Forti, 1988; Retzlaff & Bromley, 1991; Svanum & Ehrmann, 1992). These studies are all based on the assumption that some number of independent alcoholic subtypes exist, with each subtype characterized by a different etiology and a unique symptom pattern. Investigations in this area have obtained mixed results. Some studies were able to identify a "dependent subcategory" of alcoholics (Poldrugo & Forti, 1988; Retzlaff & Bromley, 1991) whose members showed a unique pattern of traits and symptoms. However, other similar studies were unable to identify a distinct subcategory of dependent alcoholic patients (Corbisiero & Reznikoff, 1991; McMahon et al., 1991; Svanum & Ehrmann, 1992).

## DEPENDENCY AND SMOKING

A number of studies support the psychoanalytic hypothesis that dependency should be associated with elevated rates of cigarette smoking (Fisher & Fisher, 1975; Jacobs et al., 1965, 1966; Jacobs & Spilken, 1971; Kimeldorf & Gewitz, 1966; Kline & Storey, 1980; Veldman & Brown, 1969). Not only do cigarette smokers obtain significantly higher dependency scores than nonsmokers (Jacobs et al., 1965, 1966; Veldman & Brown, 1969), but studies have also demonstrated that there is a significant positive correlation between level of dependency and smoking frequency (Jacobs & Spilken, 1971; Kline & Storey, 1980). Furthermore, the dependency–smoking relationship has been observed in high school (Jacobs et al., 1965), college (Veldman & Brown, 1969), and community samples (Fisher & Fisher, 1975). A variety of dependency measures and indices of smoking behavior have been employed in these studies, generally yielding consistent results.

Vaillant (1980) further found that level of dependency assessed at age 20 predicted subsequent smoking frequency in a sample of 184 male college graduates. Vaillant's results suggest that dependency actually predisposes individuals to cigarette smoking, rather than being a correlate or consequence of smoking behavior. Because Vaillant's longitudinal sample included only men, however, the degree to which dependency predisposes women to smoke remains unexamined.

Vaillant's (1980) results are consistent with the psychoanalytic hypothesis that dependent individuals tend to rely on "oral" (i.e., food- and mouth-related) activities to cope with anxiety, but a plausible alternative interpretation of these results is that the increased rates of cigarette smoking observed in the dependent men in Vaillant's sample reflect dependent individuals' susceptibility to interpersonal influence. Specifically, it may be that the dependent men in Vaillant's sample were more strongly influenced than were nondependent men by peer pressure to smoke during late adolescence. In this context, it is noteworthy that the subjects in Vaillant's sample typically initiated smoking during the 1950s and early 1960s, before strong cautionary messages regarding the dangers of cigarette smoking were commonplace. Today, an adolescent considering whether or not to smoke is confronted with (at least) two conflicting messages. One message comes from those peers who may encourage the individual to smoke in order to "fit in." An opposing message comes from the Surgeon General and other figures of authority (e.g., teachers), who strongly discourage cigarette smoking.

Thus, the social pressures surrounding cigarette smoking have changed considerably since the subjects in Vaillant's (1980) sample made their initial decisions regarding whether or not to smoke. Interestingly, given the dependent individual's desire to please figures of authority rather than peers (Bornstein et al., 1987), and the strong antismoking messages conveyed by figures of authority today, it is entirely possible that a longitudinal study of the dependency–smoking link involving today's college students would yield precisely the opposite results from those obtained by Vaillant.

The results of one experiment (Fisher & Fisher, 1975) suggest that dependency plays a role in predicting smokers' responses to cigarette deprivation. Fisher and Fisher utilized the HIT to assess dependency in a mixed-sex sample of heavy smokers (i.e., adults who reported smoking more than 30 cigarettes per day). Not surprisingly, the heavy smokers who composed Fisher and Fisher's sample showed elevated HIT dependency scores. Nonetheless, Fisher and Fisher divided their subjects into high- and low-dependent groups based on the mean HIT dependency score in this sample. Half the subjects in each group then underwent 2 hours of cigarette deprivation, while the remaining subjects were allowed to smoke as much as they wanted for the same 2-hour period. At the end of 2 hours, several measures of somatic symptoms and body image distortion were administered to all subjects. Only those subjects in the dependent/deprived group showed significantly elevated levels of somatic symptoms and body image aberration; subjects in the other three groups did not differ on either of these variables. Apparently, smoking deprivation produces stronger negative effects on body image and somatic symptomatology in dependent than in nondependent cigarette smokers.

Fisher and Fisher's (1975) results are consistent with Bornstein et al.'s (1988b) finding that dependency is associated with body image aberration and distortion in college students (Experiment 1) and psychiatric inpatients (Experiment 2). Furthermore, Fisher and Fisher's findings suggest that dependency may play a role in propagating tobacco addiction, since the somatic symptoms reported by the dependent/deprived subjects in Fisher and Fisher's study were typically highly aversive (e.g., headache, dizziness, nausea). In this respect, Fisher and Fisher's (1975) findings dovetail with those of Spolter et al. (1978) regarding alcoholic recidivism. Perhaps dependency predicts recidivism following cessation of heavy tobacco use as well as predicting recidivism following cessation of heavy drinking.

One other finding from research on dependency and smoking is noteworthy in the present context. In addition to assessing the dependency–smoking relationship, Jacobs and Spilken (1971) examined differences in parental perceptions in heavy smokers versus nonsmokers from their sample of male college students. Relative to nonsmokers, the smokers in Jacobs and Spilken's sample described their mothers as cold, harsh, demanding, and overcontrolling. Jacobs and Spilken's findings regarding the smoking–parental perceptions relationship parallel the results obtained in studies of the dependency–parental perceptions relationship (e.g., Bornstein et al., 1986), wherein dependency was found to be associated with perceptions of the mother as cold, punitive, and overcontrolling.

## DEPENDENCY AND SUBSTANCE USE DISORDERS

The theoretical link between dependency and opiate or cocaine use is more tenuous than the theoretical link between dependency and those substance use disorders that have an obvious "oral" component (i.e., smoking and drinking). However, Blatt, Rounsaville, Eyre, and Wilber (1984) provided a nice summary of the psychoanalytic view regarding the connection between dependency needs and substance use disorders. Blatt et al. (1984) suggested that these addictive disorders reflect the drug-using individual's

> desire to establish a symbiotic relatedness with the maternal object through substance use. The drug serves as a replacement for the failure to achieve a basic sense of relatedness with a nurturing, loving mother. . . . The drug is used to satisfy primitive oral cravings and to ward off depression related to intense feelings of helplessness and dependency. (p. 343)

Needless to say, social learning theorists take a very different view of the dependency–addiction relationship. The social learning view of drug addiction includes two related components. First, drug addiction reflects a simple conditioning process wherein a new pattern of behavior (i.e., habitual drug use) is acquired because it is an effective means of obtaining rewards, at least in the short term. Of course, once the addiction is well established, drug use comes to be driven by punishment avoidance (i.e., avoidance of withdrawal symptoms) in addition to pleasure seeking. Furthermore, to the extent that a drug comes to be associated with tension reduction and pain reduction, the drug will function much as did the primary caretaker of infancy—that is, as a kind of secondary reinforcer. Thus, the same kind of conditioning/learning sequence that established and maintained the infantile dependency relationship may establish and maintain drug dependency.

Blatt et al. (1984) conducted the most extensive and well-designed study of the dependency–substance use relationship. Blatt et al. compared the DEQ dependency scores of matched mixed-sex samples of opiate addicts ($n = 47$), nonopiate-addicted polydrug abusers ($n = 39$), and nondrug-using psychiatric control patients ($n = 197$). Subjects in the two drug abuse groups were undergoing voluntary treatment for their drug problems at the time that data were collected. This study had two important strengths. First, subjects came from a variety of ethnic and socioeconomic backgrounds.

Consequently, Blatt et al.'s (1984) findings may be generalized to various segments of the population. Second, in addition to collecting information regarding the kinds of drugs used by different subjects, Blatt et al. obtained information regarding (1) the duration of drug use and (2) the relative frequency with which subjects used different drugs. Not surprisingly, every subject in the opiate-addicted sample reported that their most frequently used drug was heroin. For poly-drug-abuse subjects, the most frequently used drugs were marijuana and alcohol.

Blatt et al. (1984) found that polydrug abusers and opiate addicts actually had significantly *lower* DEQ dependency scores than did nondrug-abusing psychiatric control patients. Dependency scores did not differ in members of the poly-drug-abuse and opiate-addicted groups. One might surmise that this finding reflects the affective and cognitive sequelae of drug addiction, since heavy drug use may mask overt dependency needs, instilling in the user a temporary (and false) sense of security and self-sufficiency. However, the fact that subjects in this study were undergoing drug abuse treatment at the time that the data were collected argues against this explanation of Blatt et al.'s findings. Moreover, Blatt et al. (1984) found no consistent relationship between level of dependency and duration of drug use in either drug-abusing group, nor was there any relationship between level of dependency and frequency of drug use in either group. Consistent with Blatt et al.'s findings, Block, Block, and Keyes (1988) also found no strong, consistent relationships between level of dependency and frequency or type of drug use in a mixed-sex sample of adolescents.

Using a very different subject sample and measure of dependency than was used by Blatt et al. (1984) or Block et al. (1988), Wallot and Lambert (1984) compared dependency levels in drug-abusing Canadian physicians who used one drug exclusively ($n = 16$) and those who used multiple drugs ($n = 21$). All of the physician drug users in this sample were undergoing mandatory treatment for drug abuse under the auspices of an impaired practitioner program instituted by the Quebec Board of Physicians. Data were collected from treatment (i.e., chart) records. In contrast to the findings of Blatt et al. (1984), Wallot and Lambert found that a significantly higher proportion of the poly-drug-abusing group than the single-drug-use group manifested "clinically significant passive-dependent personality traits." While only 6% of the single-drug-use group showed passive-dependent personality traits, 24% of the poly-drug-use group exhibited these traits.

Unfortunately, one important methodological limitation of Wallot and Lambert's (1984) study makes their results difficult to interpret. In this investigation, the clinicians who kept chart records were not blind to the drug-use status of the physician/patients. Thus, it is possible that clinicians' ratings of "passive dependency" were based in part on knowledge of the physician/patients' patterns of drug use, artificially inflating the observed relationship between these two variables.

Overall, the most consistent (and informative) results in this area have come from studies that compared the prevalence of different personality disorder symptoms in samples of drug-abusing individuals. To date, 10 studies have assessed the prevalence of different personality disorders in samples of drug abusers. In three of these investigations, personality disorder symptoms were assessed via the MCMI (Calsyn & Saxon, 1990; Craig, 1988; Marsh, Stile, Stoughton, & Trout-Landen, 1988). In the other seven investigations, personality disorder symptoms were assessed via a structured clinical interview (Khantzian & Treece, 1985; Kosten, Rounsaville, & Kleber, 1982; Nace, Davis, & Gaspari, 1991; Rounsaville, Rosenberger, Wilber, Weissman, & Kleber, 1980; Rounsaville, Weissman, Kleber, & Wilber, 1982; Weiss, Mirin, Michael, & Sollogub, 1986; Zimmerman & Coryell, 1989).[3] Because information regarding a variety of personality traits and personality disorder symptoms were collected in these studies, the results of these studies allow the specificity of the dependency–substance use relationship to be assessed directly.

The central findings of these 10 investigations are summarized in Table 6.1, which lists (1) the dependency measure used in each study; (2) the types of subjects examined in each study; (3) the percentage of subjects in each investigation that received DPD diagnoses; and (4) those Axis II diagnoses that were more prevalent than DPD in each sample. As Table 6.1 shows, a small to moderate proportion of the subjects showed clinically significant DPD symptomatology in most of these studies. There is some indication that opiate users may receive higher proportions of DPD diagnoses than do cocaine users or poly-drug users, but this trend is due primarily to the unusually high percentage of opiate users who received DPD diagnoses in Marsh et al.'s (1988) investigation. Not surprisingly, studies using the MCMI yielded much higher rates of DPD (and other Axis II disorders) than did studies that used clinical interviews to derive diagnoses. This pattern of results is consistent with recent suggestions that the MCMI and other questionnaire measures (e.g., the PDQ-R) may be overly lenient in assessing personality disorder symptomatology, yielding a substantial number of false positive diagnoses (Widiger, Williams, Spitzer, & Frances, 1985).

It is important to note that—as the last column in Table 6.1 shows—in all 10 of these investigations, other personality disorders (e.g., antisocial, narcissistic, borderline, histrionic) were more prevalent among the drug-abusing subjects than was DPD. Calsyn, Saxon, and Daisy (1991) also found that other personality disorders were significantly more prevalent than was DPD in a sample of drug-abusing subjects, although Calsyn et al.

**TABLE 6.1. Axis II Diagnoses in Drug-Using Subjects**

| Study | DPD measure | Subjects | Percentage of subjects receiving DPD diagnoses | Axis II disorders more prevalent than DPD |
|---|---|---|---|---|
| Calsyn & Saxon (1990) | MCMI | Opiate users | 19 | Narcissistic (36%) Antisocial (28%) |
| | MCMI | Cocaine users | 11 | Narcissistic (36%) Antisocial (28%) |
| Craig (1988) | MCMI | Opiate users | 16 | Antisocial (22%) Narcissistic (18%) |
| Khantzian & Treece (1985) | Clinical interview | Opiate users | 4 | Antisocial (53%) Avoidant (7%) |
| Kosten et al. (1982) | Clinical interview | Opiate users | 4 | Antisocial (55%) Borderline (12%) Histrionic (5%) |
| Marsh et al. (1988) | MCMI | Opiate users | 29 | Narcissistic (38%) Histrionic (34%) Antisocial (32%) |
| Nace et al. (1991) | Clinical interview | Polydrug users | 7 | Borderline (30%) Paranoid (13%) Histrionic (11%) |
| Rounsaville et al. (1980) | Clinical interview | Polydrug users | 2 | Borderline (3%) |
| Rounsaville et al. (1982) | Clinical interview | Opiate users | <5 | Antisocial (26%) |
| Weiss et al. (1986) | Clinical interview | Cocaine users | 3 | Borderline (27%) Narcissistic (23%) Histrionic (17%) |
| Zimmerman & Coryell (1989) | Clinical interview | Polydrug users | 3 | Antisocial (23%) Histrionic (12%) Schizotypal (10%) Borderline (7%) Avoidant (7%) |

*Note.* Rounsaville et al. (1982) indicated only that less than 5% of subjects in their sample received DPD diagnoses.

(1991) did not report separate prevalence rates for different disorders in this investigation. Thus, although some studies in this area suggest that dependent traits may be associated with substance use disorders (Wallot & Lambert, 1984), this relationship is neither strong nor specific. Substance abusers show high levels of a variety of personality disorder traits and symptoms, including—but not limited to—those associated with DPD.

## DEPENDENCY, OBESITY, AND EATING DISORDERS

A central tenet of classical psychoanalytic theory is that the dependent person will be preoccupied with food and eating as a means of obtaining security and nurturance (see Chapter 1 for a detailed discussion of this hypothesis). As Bornstein and Greenberg (1991) noted, the psychoanalytic model suggests that for the dependent individual, "food has tremendous symbolic importance, serving not only as sustenance, but also as a means of indirectly recapturing early feelings of security and connectedness with the primary caretaker" (p. 148). Thus, psychoanalytic theory hypothesizes that dependency should be associated with risk for obesity, and possibly with increased risk for other eating disorders (i.e., anorexia and bulimia) as well (see Bruch, 1973). Studies in these two areas will be considered separately.

### Obesity

Several studies have found that obese subjects obtain significantly higher scores than do normal-weight subjects on a variety of dependency measures (Friedman, 1959; Masling et al., 1967; Mills & Cunningham, 1988; Weiss & Masling, 1970). In addition, there has been at least one cross-cultural replication of the dependency–obesity relationship: Masling et al. (1967) and Weiss and Masling (1970) obtained very similar results in samples of American outpatients (Masling et al.) and Israeli inpatients (Weiss & Masling) undergoing treatment for obesity. In both studies, obese subjects had significantly higher dependency scores than normal-weight subjects. In contrast to the positive findings obtained by Masling et al. and others, three experiments reported negative results in this area, finding no relationship between dependency and obesity (Black, Goldstein, & Mason, 1992; Bornstein & Greenberg, 1991; Keith & Vandenberg, 1974).

Unfortunately, there are some methodological problems with studies of the dependency–obesity link. For example, several investigations (e.g., Friedman, 1959; Mills & Cunningham, 1988) did not control for potential confounding variables (e.g., overall level of psychopathology), so that observed dependency–obesity relationships in these investigations might reflect—in whole or in part—the effects of these other variables. In addition, researchers examining the dependency–obesity link generally have not distinguished subjects whose weight problems have a physiological (e.g., glandular) cause from subjects whose obesity is purely "psychological" (i.e., behavioral). Thus, the obese subjects in these studies were not homogeneous with respect to the etiology of their weight problems. Finally, as Masling and Schwartz (1979) noted, most studies in this area did not eliminate completely the possible effects of experimenter bias on observed dependency–obesity relationships. Examiners administering the ROD and other widely used projective dependency measures typically were not blind to the status of subjects in different groups (i.e., obese vs. normal weight). Thus, it is possible that examiners who were aware of the experimental hypothesis somehow encouraged obese and normal-weight subjects to respond differently on projective dependency measures.

Consistent with this hypothesis, all studies that produced positive results in this area utilized projective measures of dependency (i.e., the ROD, TAT, or Blacky test). However, of the three studies reporting nonsignificant results, one (Bornstein & Greenberg, 1991) used a projective measure and the other two (Black et al., 1992; Keith & Vandenberg, 1974) utilized self-report measures. Furthermore, the Rorschach examiners in Bornstein and Greenberg's (1991) study were blind to the experimental hypotheses throughout the testing procedures, while in all studies of the dependency–obesity link that obtained positive results, examiners were aware of the experimental hypotheses. Thus, findings to date may well be due more to experimenters' expectations than to a real dependency–obesity relationship. In fact, Masling and Schwartz (1979) noted that when experimenters' expectations were assessed directly, they were found to have a stronger effect on the dependency–obesity relationship than did the status (i.e., obese vs. normal weight) of the subjects being tested.

Only two studies (Marshall & Neill, 1977; McCully, Glucksman, & Hirsch, 1968) have gone beyond simply assessing the relationship between dependency and obesity. McCully et al. (1968) performed a within-subjects analysis comparing ROD scores in a small ($n = 6$) sample of obese inpatients: (1) before weight-reduction treatment and (2) after successful treatment (when all six patients' weights had returned to the normal range). They found that ROD scores showed no significant change over the course of the study, and interpreted these findings to suggest that dependency was not simply a correlate of the patients' obese status. Unfortunately, the sample in McCully et al.'s (1968) study was extremely small, and because all patients underwent "successful" treatment, it is impossible to know how their ROD scores might have changed following unsuccessful treatment for obesity. Furthermore, when Marshall and Neill (1977) assessed changes in overt dependent behaviors in a sample of 12 obese patients following successful intestinal-bypass surgery, they found a significant decrease in dependent behaviors following the bypass procedure (when the patients' weights had returned to the normal range). Thus, Marshall and Neill's (1977) results are inconsistent with those of McCully et al., (1968) and suggest that dependency might be a correlate or consequence of obesity.

## Eating Disorders

There have been at least 11 studies to date examining the relationship of dependency and eating disorders (i.e., anorexia and bulimia) in female psychiatric inpatients, outpatients, and college students (Bornstein & Greenberg, 1991; Jacobson & Robins, 1989; Lenihan & Kirk, 1990; Levin & Hyler, 1986; Pendleton, Tisdale, & Marler, 1991; Strauss & Ryan, 1987; Tisdale, Pendleton, & Marler, 1990; Wold, 1983; Wonderlich, Swift, Slotnick, & Goodman, 1990; Yager, Landsverk, Edelstein, & Hyler, 1989; Zimmerman & Coryell, 1989). These investigations produced stronger and more consistent results than did studies examining the dependency–obesity link.

Bornstein and Greenberg's (1991) investigation is typical of studies in this area. Bornstein and Greenberg compared the ROD scores of obese ($n =$ 18), eating-disordered ($n = 16$), and noneating-disordered, normal-weight female psychiatric inpatients ($n = 17$). Subjects in the three groups were matched on age, marital status, years of education, WAIS-R score, and number and type of psychiatric diagnoses. ROD scores were derived from Rorschach protocols that had been administered by clinical psychology interns blind to the hypotheses of the study. Although Bornstein and Greenberg found no difference between obese and control subjects' dependency scores (this finding is discussed earlier), the eating-disordered subjects in Bornstein and Greenberg's sample obtained significantly higher ROD scores than did subjects in the other two groups. In fact, eating-disordered subjects produced nearly three times as much dependent Rorschach imagery as obese subjects, and twice as much dependent imagery as control subjects.

Similar findings were reported by Yager et al. (1989), who assessed the dependency–eating disorders relationship in a sample of 628 female psychiatric inpatients. Yager et al. (1989) compared PDQ-R dependency scores (Hyler et al., 1988) in anorexic ($n = 15$), bulimic ($n = 300$), and non-eating-disordered control subjects ($n = 313$). Consistent with the findings of Bornstein and Greenberg (1991), Yager et al. found that both anorexic and bulimic subjects obtained dependency scores that were approximately twice as great as the dependency scores obtained by control subjects. Along similar lines, Tisdale et al. (1990) and Pendleton et al. (1991) found that bulimic female outpatients obtained significantly higher MCMI dependency scores (Millon, 1987) than did matched samples of non-eating-disordered female outpatients and nonclinical control subjects. Strauss and Ryan (1987), Wold (1983), and Zimmerman and Coryell (1989) reported similar results in samples of psychiatric inpatients and outpatients.

Similar findings were also obtained by Jacobson and Robins (1989), who assessed the relationship between level of dependency and amount of eating-disorder symptomatology in a sample of 330 undergraduate women. As predicted, women with high levels of eating-disorder symptomatology obtained significantly higher dependency scores than did women with low levels of eating-disorder symptomatology. Jacobson and Robins' results are consistent with those of Pendleton et al. (1991), Strauss and Ryan (1987), Tisdale et al. (1990), Yager et al. (1989), Wold (1983), Zimmerman and Coryell (1989), and Bornstein and Greenberg (1991), despite the fact that Jacobson and Robins assessed subsyndromal symptom levels while the other studies employed clinical subjects manifesting full-blown Axis I disorders.

Wonderlich et al. (1990) took a slightly different approach to this issue, assessing the degree to which symptoms of various DSM-III-R personality disorders were present in members of a sample of 46 eating-disordered female psychiatric inpatients. The advantage of Wonderlich et al.'s approach is that it allowed the specificity of the dependency–eating disorders relationship to be assessed directly. Wonderlich et al. (1990) found that DPD symptoms were among the most prevalent personality disorder symptoms in members of this sample. However, DPD symptoms were not significantly more prevalent than the symptoms of several other personality disorders in these inpatient subjects. Specifically, 32% of the women in Wonderlich et al.'s (1990) eating-disordered sample met the DSM-III-R criteria for DPD, while 32% met the criteria for avoidant personality disorder, 25% met the criteria for borderline personality disorder, 23% met the criteria for histrionic personality disorder, and 18% met the criteria for obsessive–compulsive personality disorder. Levin and Hyler (1986) also found that other personality disorders were at least as common as DPD in a sample of 24 eating-disordered women.

Thus, research examining the dependency–eating disorders relationship may be summarized as follows. Clearly, eating-disordered women show higher levels of dependency than do noneating-disordered control subjects. However, the causal relationship of dependency and eating disorders remains unexamined, and recent studies suggest that other personality traits (e.g., avoidant traits) might also be associated with anorexia and bulimia.

Two other investigations are worth mentioning briefly in the context of research on the dependency–eating disorders relationship. Lacey, Coker, and Birtchnell (1986) and Pyle, Mitchell, and Eckert (1981) both found that experiences of interpersonal loss and rejection were among the most common precipitants of eating disorders in women. Although subjects' level of dependency was not assessed in these studies, Lacey et al.'s (1986) and Pyle et al.'s (1981) findings regarding interpersonal stressors as precipitants of eating disorders parallel the results of several studies (e.g., Hammen et al., 1985, 1989a, 1989b) which found that interpersonal stressors were a significant factor in the onset of depressive episodes in dependent individuals.

## DISENTANGLING THE DEPENDENCY–PSYCHOPATHOLOGY RELATIONSHIP

Because the dependency–psychopathology relationship is complex and differs for different types of psychological disorders, it is worthwhile to briefly review the results obtained in this area. Table 6.2 summarizes in general

**TABLE 6.2. Summary of Dependency–Psychopathology Relationships**

| Disorder | Dependency–psychopathology relationship |
|---|---|
| Depression | Strong correlational evidence for a dependency–depression link<br>Dependency and depression levels covary in longitudinal and experimental studies<br>Dependency and interpersonal stress combine to predict the onset of depression |
| Phobias | Strong correlational evidence for dependency–school phobia and dependency–agoraphobia links<br>Specificity of the dependency–school phobia and dependency–agoraphobia relationships remains open to question |
| Alcoholism | Increases in dependency follow the onset of alcoholism |
| Smoking | Dependency predicts the onset of cigarette smoking<br>Dependency predicts response to cigarette deprivation in smokers |
| Substance use disorders | Evidence for a relationship between dependency and substance disorders is weak<br>Opiate users may show higher dependency levels than do cocaine or poly-drug users |
| Obesity and eating disorders | Dependency–obesity studies have produced inconclusive results<br>Strong correlational evidence for a dependency–eating disorders link<br>Specificity of the dependency–eating disorders link is questionable<br>Causal relationship of dependency and eating disorders remains unexplored |

terms the findings obtained thus far regarding the relationship of dependency to the six categories of psychopathology discussed in this chapter. As this table shows, dependency predicts the onset of certain disorders (i.e., depression, tobacco addiction) and follows the onset of others (i.e., alcoholism). For phobias and eating disorders, correlational evidence confirms that dependency is associated with elevated symptom levels and with increased incidences of these disorders. However, studies conducted to date have provided no information regarding the causal relationship between dependency and these two types of psychopathology. Finally, research regarding the dependency–obesity link is methodologically flawed and inconclusive. Studies suggest that there is little if any relationship between dependency and substance use disorders.

Not surprisingly, two methodological limitations that have traditionally hindered studies of personality–psychopathology relationships also characterize studies of the dependency–psychopathology relationship. First, researchers have done a much better job exploring the association of dependency with particular forms of psychopathology than they have in demonstrating the causal relationship between these variables. Second, with a few noteworthy exceptions, researchers have failed to address the specificity of particular dependency–psychopathology links. It would be an overstatement to suggest that the dependency–psychopathology relationship is completely nonspecific. However, it does seem that when self-report data are collected and correlational designs are used, dependency is associated with a wide variety of psychological disorders.

Bornstein and Johnson's (1990) findings regarding the relationship of PDQ-R dependency scores (Hyler et al., 1988) to SCL-90 psychopathology scores (Derogatis et al., 1973) illustrate the broad range of psychopathologies that are found to be associated with dependency in correlational studies using self-report measures. The central findings from this investigation are summarized in Table 6.3. As this table shows, significant correlations between PDQ-R dependency scores and SCL-90 psychopathology scores were obtained in every area assessed (column 1). When the effect of social desirability on reporting of psychological symptoms was taken into account (column 2), dependency scores were still significantly correlated with scores on seven of nine specific dimensions of psychopathology. Furthermore, the significant correlations between PDQ-R dependency scores and scores on the General Symptom Index and Positive Symptom Total scales of the SCL-90 indicate that dependent subjects in this study reported experiencing a large number (and wide range) of psychological symptoms. Similar results were subsequently obtained by Nakao et al., (1992), who found that MCMI dependency scores were positively correlated with total number of Axis II symptoms ($r = .47$), and with scores on the DSM-III-R Axis V Global Assessment of Functioning (GAF) scale ($r = -.31$), in a mixed-sex sample of Japanese psychiatric outpatients.

**TABLE 6.3. Summary of Observed Dependency–Psychopathology Relationships in Bornstein and Johnson's Study**

| | Dependency–psychopathology correlation | |
| --- | --- | --- |
| SCL-90 scale | Uncorrected | Controlling for social desirability score |
| Somatization | .24* | .15 |
| Obsessive–compulsive | .37*** | .27* |
| Interpersonal sensitivity | .67**** | .59**** |
| Depression | .46**** | .41*** |
| Anxiety | .32* | .24* |
| Hostility | .29* | .19 |
| Phobia | .35** | .30* |
| Paranoia | .33* | .25* |
| Psychoticism | .36** | .31* |
| General symptom index | .45**** | .37*** |
| Positive symptom total | .44**** | .35** |

*Note.* n of subjects = 45 (26 women and 19 men). Partial correlations were computed controlling for Crowne–Marlowe (1964) social desirability scores. General symptom index and positive symptom total scores reflect the degree to which subjects acknowledged experiencing a wide variety of psychological symptoms.
*$p$ < .05. **$p$ < .01. ***$p$ < .005. ****$p$ < .001.
Adapted from Bornstein and Johnson (1990, Table 1). © 1990 by Select Press. Adapted by permission of the publisher.

Thus, three issues will continue to confront dependency–psychopathology researchers during the coming years. First, researchers must continue to disentangle the causal relationship between dependency and various dimensions of psychological symptomatology. To this end, a longitudinal study comparing the prevalence of various psychological disorders in dependent versus nondependent individuals is needed. Second, researchers must address more directly questions regarding the specificity of observed dependency–psychopathology relationships. It may be that a large-scale multicenter epidemiological study will be required to address this question conclusively. Third, researchers should explore more fully the possible effects of dependency on treatment outcome. Preliminary results in this area suggest that dependency plays a role in determining the outcome of psychological and pharmacological treatment for phobias (Mavissakalian & Hamann, 1987), and may also predict responsivity to treatment for alcoholism (Spolter, 1978) and tobacco addiction (Fisher & Fisher, 1975). Continued exploration of the dependency–treatment efficacy relationship will likely yield practical benefits as well as theoretical insights.

What are the implications of the findings reviewed in this chapter for the psychoanalytic and social learning theories of dependency? In a sense, findings regarding the dependency–psychopathology relationship parallel earlier findings regarding the etiology of dependency: They are consistent with the social learning model but do not allow the psychoanalytic model to be ruled out definitively. As discussed in Chapter 1, the key difference between the psychoanalytic and social learning models with respect to psychopathology is that the psychoanalytic model hypothesizes that dependency should be associated with preoccupation with "oral" activities (e.g., eating, drinking, smoking) as a means of coping with anxiety, while the social learning view does not predict that dependent individuals should engage in these activities more frequently than nondependent individuals. An additional hypothesis is implicit in the psychoanalytic prediction regarding the relationship of dependency to "oral" psychopathologies: Since dysfunctional eating, drinking, and smoking behaviors are all rooted in underlying, unresolved oral dependency needs, these behaviors should covary within individuals. In other words, individuals with one type of "oral" psychopathology should be at increased risk for other theoretically-related "oral" disorders.

Results in this area are mixed. Consistent with the psychoanalytic view, dependency predicts the likelihood of cigarette smoking in men and furthermore appears to play a role in determining individuals' responses to smoking cessation. Similarly, dependency is associated with eating disorders in women. However, the finding that dependency does not predict risk for alcoholism is inconsistent with the psychoanalytic view. Unfortunately, studies of dependency and obesity are so flawed methodologically that the relationship between these variables remains open to question.

Findings regarding the covariation of dysfunctional eating, drinking, and smoking behaviors are also mixed, although they are generally inconsistent with the psychoanalytic view. The most comprehensive study of this issue was conducted by Beckwith (1986), who examined the relationship of dysfunctional eating, drinking, and cigarette smoking behaviors in a sample of 766 20–30-year-old Australian women. Beckwith found that indices of dysfunctional eating and drinking behaviors were unrelated in her female subjects ($r = .04$), as were indices of dysfunctional eating and smoking behaviors ($r = -.01$). However, there was a significant positive correlation between smoking and drinking levels in these subjects ($r = .38$).

The inconsistent relationship between dependency and risk for psychopathologies that have a clear oral component—coupled with Beckwith's (1986) mixed results regarding the covariation of eating, drinking, and smoking behaviors in normal subjects—calls into question the psychoanalytic hypothesis that there exists a recognizable cluster of "oral dependent" psychopathologies. These results therefore raise a fundamental question regarding the psychoanalytic model of dependency: Is dependency actually associated with preoccupation with food- and mouth-related activities, as the psychoanalytic model suggests?

In general, findings in this area do not support the psychoanalytic view. Although some factor-analytic and correlational studies have found that level of dependency is positively correlated with degree of preoccupation with food- and mouth-related activities (Beller, 1957; Jamison & Comrey, 1968; Mills & Cunningham, 1988), other similar studies found no relationship between these variables (Kline & Storey, 1980). Furthermore, two particularly well-designed investigations produced negative results regarding the hypothesized orality–dependency link. First, Shilkret and Masling (1981) found a nonsignificant relationship ($r = -.06$) between scores on the Rorschach "dependency" and "food- and mouth-related activities" scales in a mixed-sex sample of undergraduates. Second, Bornstein and Greenberg (1991) found a nonsignificant relationship between Rorschach dependency and food/mouth scores in a sample of female psychiatric inpatients. If future studies confirm that dependency and preoccupation with food and eating are in fact orthogonal traits, this would contradict a central prediction made by the classical psychoanalytic model.

## NOTES

1. There have also been several studies examining possible links between dependency and suicidality. Unfortunately, these investigations produced inconsistent, inconclusive results, with some studies finding that dependent individuals are at greater risk for suicide than are nondependent individuals (e.g., Finn, 1955; Iga, 1966; Pallis & Birtchnell, 1976; Tabachnick, 1961), and other studies finding no relationship between dependency and suicidality (e.g., Lester, 1969; Overholser, Kabakoff, & Norman, 1989).

2. Cramer, Blatt, and Ford (1988) also examined the dependency–defense mechanism relationship. However, they used a very different measure of defense mechanism usage (i.e., TAT responses), and furthermore assessed different dimensions of defensive style than were assessed in the Bornstein et al. (1990) and Levit (1991) studies. Thus, it is not possible to compare directly the findings obtained in these three investigations. Cramer et al.'s results indicated that dependency was not significantly related to reliance on the defense mechanisms of projection, denial, or identification in a mixed-sex sample of psychiatric inpatients.

3. Although Alnaes and Torgerson (1988b) also assessed the prevalence of DPD in substance abusers, these data are not included in Table 6.1 because the inclusion and exclusion criteria used to select substance-abusing patients for this study were idiosyncratic in two respects. First, Alnaes and Torgerson's substance abusing sample may have included patients with alcohol and tobacco use disorders in addition to patients with "traditional" substance use disorders (e.g., cocaine abuse). Second, this sample excluded certain patients who were using drugs at the time of admission to the outpatient facility where data were collected.

# CHAPTER 7

# Dependent Personality Disorder

No review of research on the dependent personality would be complete without some discussion of Dependent Personality Disorder (DPD). However, DPD research differs from all the other research discussed in this book in one important respect: Whereas research on the developmental, social, and clinical aspects of dependency has almost invariably examined the effects of exaggerated dependency needs on some *other* dimension of behavior (e.g., interpersonal sensitivity), most studies of DPD have focused on the prevalence of this disorder in various subject groups, on the relationship of DPD to other psychological disorders, and on the reliability of DPD symptoms and diagnoses. In other words, although research on dependency has tended to focus on the connection between dependent personality traits and other aspects of behavior, DPD research has not yet gone beyond the investigation of basic diagnostic and psychometric issues. To be sure, there is ample evidence that DPD symptoms can mediate the onset and course of various Axis I disorders (see, e.g., Alnaes & Torgerson, 1988b; Bornstein & Greenberg, 1991; Corbisiero & Reznikoff, 1991; Goldberg et al., 1989; Greenberg & Bornstein, 1988b; Mavissakalian & Hamann, 1987; Millon, 1981; Nakao et al., 1992; Poldrugo & Forti, 1988). Nonetheless, we still have much to learn about the validity and utility of the DPD diagnosis.

In the following sections, I discuss research on (1) the construct validity of the DPD symptom criteria; (2) the prevalence of DPD in various subject groups; and (3) gender differences in DPD prevalence rates.

## THE CONSTRUCT VALIDITY OF THE DPD SYMPTOM CRITERIA

Despite the fact that Kraeplin (1913), Schneider (1923), Abraham (1927), Fenichel (1945), and others discussed at length the clinical implications of exaggerated dependency needs, the concept of the dependent personality received only passing mention in the DSM-I (APA, 1952). The DSM-I precursor of DPD was actually a subtype of the passive–aggressive personality, identified as the "passive–aggressive personality, passive–dependent type." These passive–dependent individuals were characterized by "helplessness, indecisiveness, and a tendency to cling to others as a dependent child to a supporting parent" (APA, 1952, p. 37). Oddly enough, the concept of the dependent personality received even less attention in the DSM-II (APA, 1968) than it had received in the DSM-I. In the DSM-II, the passive–dependent personality was relegated to a "catchall" category of "other personality disorders of specified types," a grouping that also included the "immature" personality. The DSM-II provided neither a description of the symptoms underlying passive–dependent personality disorder nor any hypotheses regarding the etiology of the disorder.

Finally, a full-fledged diagnostic category of DPD was included in both the DSM-III (APA, 1980) and DSM-III-R (APA, 1987). In the DSM-III, DPD was defined in terms of three broad (and somewhat overlapping) symptoms: (1) passivity in interpersonal relationships coupled with an inability to function independently; (2) willingness to subordinate one's own needs to those of others; and (3) lack of self-confidence. Although these symptom criteria were more specific than those described in the DSM-I (APA, 1952), they were still somewhat vague and furthermore lacked discriminant validity: Other DSM-III disorders (e.g., agoraphobia) were characterized by very similar symptom patterns.

The DSM-III-R (APA, 1987) criteria for DPD were far more detailed than were the DPD criteria promulgated in earlier versions of the DSM series. In the DSM-III-R, DPD is characterized primarily by "a pervasive pattern of dependent and submissive behavior, beginning by early adulthood and present in a variety of contexts" (APA, 1987, p. 354). This "pervasive pattern of dependent and submissive behavior" is associated with nine specific symptoms; the individual must show five or more of these symptoms to receive the DPD diagnosis. According to the DSM-III-R, the individual suffering from DPD (1) is unable to make independent decisions; (2) allows others to make important decisions for him or her; (3) has excessive fear of rejection; (4) has difficulty initiating projects or activities; (5) volunteers to perform unpleasant or demeaning tasks in order to please others; (6) feels helpless when alone; (7) feels devastated when important relationships end; (8) is preoccupied with fears of being abandoned; and (9) is easily hurt by criticism or disapproval. In effect, these nine symptoms fall into two broad areas: (1) behavioral (symptoms 1, 2, 4, and 5); and (2) affective (symptoms 3, 6, 7, 8, and 9).

Scrutiny of the DPD symptom criteria reveals one important strength and one potential problem. On the positive side, the DPD symptom criteria clearly assess dependency-related behaviors and are relatively free from attachment-related confounds. In other words, the attachment-related proximity-seeking behaviors that are assessed by some interview and behavioral measures of dependency (e.g., Beller's [1955] rating scale) are excluded from the DPD symptom criteria (although in this context it must be noted that Livesley et al. [1990] argued that DPD symptoms 6, 7, and 8 tap affective responses that are in part attachment related). The fact that DPD symptom criteria focus primarily on dependency-related behaviors and affective responses is an important strength: As noted in Chapter 2, dependency measures that assess attachment-related behaviors in addition to dependent traits do not allow researchers to distinguish dependency from insecure attachment in individual subjects.

On the negative side, the behaviors and affective responses assessed by the nine DPD symptom criteria are not completely independent. To be sure, some overlap among the criteria within any diagnostic category is to be expected (see Blashfield & Livesley, 1991; Hirschfeld, Shea, & Weise, 1991; Morey, Waugh, & Blashfield, 1985). Because different symptoms are presumed to reflect different aspects of the same syndrome, they should not be orthogonal. However, in at least two instances, different DPD symptom criteria appear to be assessing aspects of the same entity. For example, DPD symptoms 1 and 2 are very closely related, and it is difficult to imagine how a patient could exhibit one of these symptoms without showing the other one as well. Similarly, the affective reactions described in symptoms 7 and 8 appear to be assessing different dimensions of the same emotional response. To the extent that different symptom criteria tap the same affective, cognitive, or behavioral dimension (as opposed to simply covarying within subjects), individual symptom criteria lose their predictive validity. As future versions of the DSM series are constructed, it is likely that difficulties such as these will be eliminated.[1]

In addition to describing the symptoms that compose the DPD syndrome, the DSM-III-R (APA, 1987) offers some hypotheses regarding the co-occurrence of DPD with other psychological disorders. According to the DSM-III-R, DPD is frequently associated with histrionic, schizotypal, narcissistic, and avoidant personality disorders. The DSM-III-R further suggests that depression and anxiety disorders may be frequent concomitants of DPD. Not surprisingly, there have been a number of studies assessing the co-occurrence of DPD with other Axis I and Axis II diagnoses. In general, these studies support the assertions of the DSM-III-R (see Alnaes & Torgerson, 1988b, 1990; Hirschfeld et al., 1991; Hyler, Skodol, Kellman, Oldham & Rosnick, 1990; Jackson et al., 1991b; Jackson et al., 1991c; Joffe, Swinson, & Regan, 1988; Livesley, Jackson, & Schroeder, 1989; McCann, 1991; Mezzich, Fabrega, & Coffman, 1987; Morey et al., 1985; Nurnberg et al., 1991; Oldham et al., 1992; Pfohl, Corgell, Zimmerman,

& Stangl, 1986; Piersma, 1987; Pincus & Wiggins, 1990; Reich, 1987a, 1987b; 1987c; Reich et al., 1987; Torgerson & Alnaes, 1990; Widiger & Sanderson, 1987; Zimmerman & Coryell, 1989). However, these studies also suggest that DPD may be associated with a wider range of disorders than is acknowledged in the DSM-III-R.

Alnaes and Torgerson's (1988b) findings illustrate the pattern of re-sults typically obtained in studies of the DPD–Axis I disorder relationship. Alnaes and Torgerson calculated the ratio between the observed and ex-pected frequencies of each Axis I disorder in a mixed-sex sample of psy-chiatric outpatients diagnosed as having DPD and compared these pre-valence rates to those obtained in a matched mixed-sex sample of non-DPD outpatients. Alnaes and Torgerson found higher-than-expected prevalences of major depression, dysthymia, panic disorder, cyclothymia, social phobia, substance use disorder, and agoraphobia among their DPD patients. Tor-gerson and Alnaes (1990) subsequently reported similar results in an in-vestigation of the relationship between DPD and other Axis II disorders. In this study, higher-than-expected rates of avoidant, passive–aggressive, schi-zotypal, and borderline symptoms were found in psychiatric outpatients diagnosed as having DPD. Alnaes and Torgerson's (1988b, 1990) results echo Bornstein and Johnson's (1990) findings (described in detail in Chap-ter 6), which demonstrated that when dependency measures and indices of psychopathology are obtained concurrently, dependency is associated with a wide range of psychological symptoms.

Other investigators have assessed directly the construct validity of DPD symptom criteria and DPD diagnoses. In these studies, DPD diagnoses are regarded as being analogous to supra-threshold scores on a psychological test or screening inventory, while DPD symptoms are treated as test items (or subscales) that contribute to the total test score. Blashfield and Livesley (1991) discussed in detail the logic underlying these investigations, noting the parallels between psychiatric diagnoses and classification decisions that are made based on the results of traditional psychological tests. They con-cluded that in light of these parallels, the same strategies that are used to assess the construct validity of a typical objective or projective test may sometimes be used to assess the construct validity of diagnostic criteria. For example, like traditional psychological tests, diagnostic criteria should show acceptable levels of concurrent, predictive, convergent, and discriminant validity. Similarly, like projective tests, diagnostic criteria should show ac-ceptable levels of interrater reliability when interview-based measures are used to assess symptoms. Moreover, Axis II diagnoses should show high levels of test–retest reliability, even over relatively long periods, because Axis II symptoms are presumed to be characteristic of an individual's long-term functioning (see APA, 1987, 1991).

Using the logic described by Blashfield and Livesley (1991), numerous researchers have examined the construct validity of the DPD symptom criteria, producing strong findings in certain areas and weaker results in others. On the positive side, it is clear that DPD symptoms tend to co-occur within individual subjects, forming a recognizable cluster or "syndrome" (Livesley et al., 1990; Millon, 1987; Morey, 1988). Furthermore, although there is some overlap between DPD symptoms and symptoms of related Axis II disorders (e.g., avoidant personality disorder), correlational and factor analytic studies confirm that DPD symptom ratings show adequate discriminant validity (Frances & Widiger, 1987; Hirschfeld et al., 1991; McCann, 1991; Strack, Lorr, & Campbell, 1990). Moreover, McMahon et al. (1985) and Stankovic et al. (1992) found that DPD symptom ratings showed adequate test–retest stability over a 2-month period in a variety of subject groups. Along different lines, detailed information regarding inter-rater reliability in DPD diagnosis was provided by Mellsop, Varghese, Joshua, and Hicks (1982), and by Spitzer, Forman, and Nee (1979). Kappa coefficients for DPD diagnoses in the Mellsop et al. (1982) and Spitzer et al. (1979) studies were among the highest reported for Axis II personality disorders.

Although evidence supporting the internal validity of the DPD symptoms is reasonably strong, the same is not true of evidence regarding the external validity of the DPD symptom criteria. In fact, there is not a single published study wherein the relationship of DPD diagnoses to the presence of the specific traits and behaviors that make up the DSM-III-R DPD symptom criteria is assessed directly. The studies discussed in Chapters 4 and 6 do allow some conclusions to be drawn regarding the external validity of the DPD symptoms, but these conclusions must be regarded as highly tentative because the vast majority of the investigations discussed in these chapters used objective or projective dependency measures—not DPD symptoms—to select dependent individuals for study (cf. Craig, 1988; Hayward & King, 1990; Poldrugo & Forti, 1988). In any case, the results of the investigations discussed in Chapters 4 and 6 generally support the validity of DPD symptoms 1, 3, 5, 6, 7, and 9; are equivocal with respect to DPD symptoms 2 and 8; and do not support the validity of DPD symptom 4. Without question, an important task for researchers during the coming years will be to assess directly the external validity of the DPD symptom criteria that are promulgated in future versions of the DSM series.

## THE PREVALENCE OF DPD

To date, 18 studies have assessed the prevalence of DPD in various subject groups using DSM-III (APA, 1980) or DSM-III-R (APA, 1987) criteria to make DPD diagnoses.[2] These studies are listed in Table 7.1. In the majority of these investigations, diagnostic information was obtained via structured clinical interview (Alnaes & Torgerson, 1988a; Drake et al., 1988; Hayward & King, 1990; Jackson, Gazis, Rudd, & Edwards, 1991a; Jackson et al., 1991c; Nace et al., 1991; Nurnberg et al., 1991; Poldrugo & Forti, 1988; Reich, 1987b; Trull, Widiger, & Frances, 1987; Widiger, Freiman, & Bailey, 1990; Widiger & Sanderson, 1987; Zimmerman & Coryell, 1989), although in five studies diagnostic information was obtained from chart records (Kass, Spitzer, & Williams, 1983; Koenigsberg, Kaplan, Gilmore, & Cooper, 1985; Mezzich, Fabrega, & Coffman, 1987; Piersma, 1987; Stangler & Printz, 1980).

**TABLE 7.1. Prevalence of DPD in Various Subject Groups**

| Study | Sample | Proportion of Ss with DPD | | |
|---|---|---|---|---|
| | | Women | Men | Overall |
| Alnaes & Torgerson (1988a) | 298 outpatients | 48 | 46 | 47 |
| Drake et al. (1988) | 396 community subjects | — | 10 | 10 |
| Hayward & King (1990) | 45 community subjects | 0 | 0 | 0 |
| Jackson et al. (1991a) | 82 inpatients | — | — | 20 |
| Jackson et al. (1991c) | 112 inpatients | 25 | 11 | 17 |
| Kass et al. (1983) | 2,192 community subjects | 11 | 5 | 8 |
| | 531 outpatients | 9 | 4 | 7 |
| Koenigsberg et al. (1985) | 2,462 outpatients | — | — | 3 |
| Mezzich et al. (1987) | 11,292 outpatients | — | — | 2 |
| Nace et al. (1991) | 100 inpatients | — | — | 4 |
| Nurnberg et al. (1991) | 110 outpatients | — | — | 16 |
| Piersma (1987) | 151 inpatients | — | — | 6 |
| Poldrugo & Forti (1988) | 404 outpatients | — | 4 | 4 |
| Reich (1987b) | 170 outpatients | 27 | 16 | 24 |
| Stangler & Printz (1980) | 500 outpatients | 4 | 4 | 4 |
| Trull et al. (1987) | 84 inpatients | — | — | 48 |
| Widiger et al. (1990) | 50 inpatients | — | — | 51 |
| Widiger & Sanderson (1987) | 53 inpatients | — | — | 51 |
| Zimmerman & Coryell (1989) | 797 community subjects | 3 | 0 | 2 |

*Note.* All studies in this table used DSM-III or DSM-III-R criteria to diagnose DPD. Those studies wherein DPD prevalence rates are listed only in the "overall" column reported only pooled prevealence data, collapsed across gender.

Studies wherein the prevalence of DPD was calculated from non-representative subject samples (e.g., patients specifically seeking treatment for certain types of problems) (see Hyler et al., 1990; Oldham et al., 1992) were not included in Table 7.1, because inclusion of these data would have biased the base rate estimates of DPD that were obtained in studies in which unselected groups of subjects were assessed. Similarly, studies wherein the prevalence of DPD was assessed in subject samples that were selected based on the presence or absence of certain diagnoses were not included in Table 7.1 (see, e.g., Nakao et al.'s [1992] study that excluded patients with diagnoses of schizophrenia). Finally, studies wherein the prevalence of DPD was assessed via the MCMI (Millon, 1987) or by other questionnaire measures (e.g., the PDQ-R; Hyler et al., 1988) were not included in this table, because—as noted in Chapter 6—questionnaire measures of personality disorder symptomatology appear to be overly lenient in identifying DPD subjects, yielding a substantial number of false positive diagnoses and artificially inflating DPD prevalence rates (see Jackson et al., 1991a; Piersma, 1987; Reich, 1987a; Torgerson & Alnaes, 1990; Widiger et al., 1985).

Table 7.1 lists the sample size, the type of subjects used (i.e., psychiatric inpatients, psychiatric outpatients, or community subjects), and the percentage of subjects receiving a DPD diagnosis in each of the 18 studies listed earlier. As Table 7.1 (column 3) shows, there was wide variation in the percentage of subjects receiving a DPD diagnosis in different studies. The prevalence of DPD in these investigations ranged from a low of 0% (Hayward & King, 1990) to a high of 51% (Widiger & Sanderson, 1987). It was possible to calculate the overall prevalence of DPD across all the studies listed in Table 7.1 by pooling the data from these investigations. There were a total of 20,729 subjects in the 18 studies listed in this table. Of these, 1,089 subjects (5% of the total sample) received a DPD diagnosis.

Further information regarding this issue can be obtained by calculating the prevalence of DPD in different subject groups. A total of 632 psychiatric inpatients were included in the studies listed in Table 7.1. Of these, 134 (21%) received a DPD diagnosis. The proportion of outpatient subjects who received a DPD diagnosis was considerably lower (577 out of 15,947 subjects, or 4% of the total outpatient group). Finally, of the 4,150 community subjects included in these studies, 368 (9%) received a DPD diagnosis.

These results suggest that DPD is quite prevalent among psychiatric inpatients, somewhat less prevalent in nonclinical subjects, and least prevalent in psychiatric outpatients. These data further indicate that the overall incidence of DPD is comparable to the base rate of the most prevalent Axis I disorders (see Robins et al., 1984). For example, Robins et al. reported that lifetime prevalence rates for phobias in various samples of community subjects ranged from 1% to 10% (depending on the severity of the phobic symptoms, the degree of impairment associated with the symptoms, and the characteristics of the sample being studied). Lifetime prevalence rates for major depression in Robins et al.'s (1984) community samples ranged from 1% to just over 10% (depending on the age and socioeconomic status of the subjects being examined).

Similarly, the results of studies that compare directly the prevalence of different personality disorders within a single sample indicate that DPD is among the most common Axis II disorders in both clinical and nonclinical subjects (Alnaes & Torgerson, 1988a, 1988b; Antoni, Levine, Tischer, Green, & Millon, 1987; Drake et al., 1988; Jackson et al., 1991a, 1991c; Kass et al., 1983; Koenigsberg et al., 1985; Stangler & Printz, 1980). For example, in Kass et al.'s (1983) community sample of 2,712 subjects, DPD had the highest prevalence rate of any Axis II personality disorder (borderline, obsessive–compulsive, passive–aggressive, and histrionic personality disorders had slightly lower prevalence rates). A similar pattern of results was obtained in Kass et al.'s outpatient sample, except that in this sample borderline personality disorder was somewhat more prevalent than DPD, especially among men.

Returning to the studies listed in Table 7.1, it is noteworthy (and surprising) to find that DPD appears to be more prevalent in nonclinical subjects than in psychiatric outpatients. In the absence of data comparing the degree of social and occupational impairment in DPD and non-DPD subjects, it is impossible to draw firm conclusions regarding the implications of this result. However, three explanations for this finding seem plausible. First, it is possible that this finding is artifactual. The vast majority of outpatient subjects in Table 7.1 came from Mezzich et al.'s (1987) investigation, which had the second-lowest DPD prevalence rate of the 18 studies listed in this table (2%). Perhaps Mezzich et al. used overly stringent criteria to make DPD diagnoses. When the proportion of outpatient subjects receiving DPD diagnoses is recalculated excluding Mezzich et al.'s sample, the base rate of DPD in outpatients becomes 8% (351 out of 4,655 patients), which is in the expected range—comparable to the base rate of DPD in community subjects, but lower than the base rate of DPD in inpatients.

Another viable explanation for the pattern of results summarized in Table 7.1 has to do with the degree of impairment associated with DPD. As noted earlier, there are no data available that address this issue directly. However, it may be that contrary to the assertions of the DSM-III-R, DPD is not associated with significant social or occupational impairment or with high levels of subjective distress. If DPD is in fact ego syntonic and does not result in markedly impaired functioning, perhaps individuals with DPD are not impelled to seek treatment for the disorder. In fact, the data summarized in Table 7.1 suggest that individuals with DPD might actually be *less* likely than non-DPD individuals to seek outpatient treatment.

Finally, it is possible that the base rate of DPD in outpatient samples is comparable to (or higher than) the base rate of DPD in nonclinical samples, but that—for any of a variety of reasons—DPD is underdiagnosed in outpatients. In other words, the relatively low base rate of DPD in outpatients relative to community subjects could be due to a substantial number of false negative DPD diagnoses among the outpatients. Perhaps DPD is underdiagnosed in outpatients because DPD symptoms are relatively subtle and easily masked by the more prominent symptoms typically associated with outpatients' presenting complaints (e.g., depression, anxiety disorders).

Of course, this hypothesis cannot account for the finding that the base rate of DPD in psychiatric inpatients is more than five times higher than the base rate of DPD in psychiatric outpatients. Surely the symptoms associated with the presenting complaints of inpatients would mask DPD symptoms at least as well as do the less serious symptoms associated with the presenting complaints of outpatients. In other words, if mild to moderate levels of depression and anxiety effectively mask DPD symptoms in psychiatric outpatients, the more severe levels of depression and anxiety that are characteristic of inpatients should mask DPD symptoms even more completely.

Thus, we must look elsewhere for clues that explain these results. One possible explanation for these findings lies in the iatrogenic effects of psychiatric hospitalization. Specifically, the very high incidence of DPD diagnoses in psychiatric inpatients could be an indirect result of the high levels of overt dependent behavior that are characteristic of hospitalized patients in general. Numerous researchers have documented the increases in dependent behavior (frequently termed "institutional dependency") that follow the initiation of inpatient treatment for psychological and medical disorders (e.g., Alsop, 1984; Barton et al., 1980; Booth, 1986; Colton, 1980; Eddington, Piper, Tanna, Hodkinson, & Salmon, 1990; Linke & Taylor, 1987). Although significant increases in patients' dependent behavior are observed after only a brief period of hospitalization, it also appears that the frequency (and intensity) of dependent behaviors increases as hospitalization continues. As Booth (1986) noted:

[T]he apathy, helplessness, withdrawal and disorientation that research has shown to be so widespread among [hospital] residents have been linked to the nature of institutional regimes. . . . As residents grow more inured to residential life, so they become more dependent on the routine imposed on their lives. (p. 418)

Perhaps the exaggerated dependent behaviors typically shown by hospitalized patients lead clinicians and clinical researchers to overdiagnose DPD in inpatients. This possibility has never been explored.

## SEX DIFFERENCES IN DPD

The studies listed in Table 7.1 allow strong conclusions to be drawn regarding sex differences in DPD. In 8 of the 18 studies listed in this table, separate estimates of the prevalence of DPD were calculated for male and female subjects. In addition, 2 studies (Drake et al., 1988; Poldrugo & Forti, 1988) used male subjects only. Pooling the data from these 10 investigations allows for an empirical analysis of sex differences in the prevalence of DPD. Of a total of 2,766 women for whom DPD base rate data are available from the studies listed in Table 7.1, 299 (11%) received a DPD diagnosis. Of 3,199 men for whom base rate data are available, 257 (8%) received a DPD diagnosis. This difference is highly significant ($\chi^2$ [1, $n$ = 5,965] = 13.53, $p$ = .0005) and suggests that the base rate of DPD is substantially higher in women than in men.

It is certainly possible that these observed sex differences in DPD reflect real base rate differences in the prevalence of this disorder. However, an equally plausible interpretation of these findings is that they are due to some type of methodological artifact (e.g., nonrepresentative sampling of subjects, problems with diagnostic reliability, examiner bias).[3] It may be possible to discover the origin of these gender differences in DPD base rates, or at least to rule out some possible causes. To begin to address this issue, a brief discussion of sources of gender differences in psychiatric diagnosis is required.

### Sources of Gender Differences in Psychiatric Diagnosis

Widiger and Spitzer (1991) discussed in detail the methodological pitfalls that can undermine research on sex differences in psychiatric diagnosis. They note that several methodological artifacts can potentially produce differential base rates of a particular disorder in men and women, even when in reality men and women show comparable base rates of the disorder in question. For example, characteristics of the setting in which base rate information is collected can influence the likelihood that sex differences in the prevalence of a disorder will be found. Thus, the patterns of sex differences obtained in samples of hospitalized VA patients may be quite different from the patterns of sex differences obtained in samples of patients at a state psychiatric hospital or a private facility. Widiger and Spitzer refer to this as "sampling sex bias."

Alternatively, bias on the part of clinicians might produce differential rates of false positive (or false negative) diagnoses for a particular disorder in men and women, leading to an overestimate of sex differences in the prevalence of that disorder. In Widiger and Spitzer's (1991) scheme, this would represent a form of "diagnostic sex bias." With respect to DPD, it is possible that patients' sex-role characteristics bias clinicians' and clinical researchers' judgments, with DPD diagnoses made in part on the basis of feminine attitudes, feelings, and behaviors described or exhibited by a patient. In other words, in the minds of clinicians and clinical researchers, femininity may be so strongly associated with dependency that when a person appears feminine, dependency is "automatically" (i.e., unconsciously and reflexively) attributed to that individual. Ashmore's (1981) finding that dependency is a central characteristic of most people's conceptions of femininity supports this hypothesis (see also Broverman et al., 1972; Cadbury, 1991; Maccoby & Jacklin, 1974; Yeger & Miezitis, 1985).

A third possible source of bias in psychiatric diagnosis lies not in characteristics of the setting or the diagnostician, but in the nature of the diagnostic criteria themselves. It is possible that the symptom criteria for a particular disorder are constructed in such a way that the disorder will inevitably be over- or underdiagnosed in men or women. If, for example, extreme menstrual discomfort was considered a symptom of a particular disorder, and there was no comparable symptom of the disorder that could potentially be exhibited by men, inclusion of this symptom would most likely result in overdiagnosis of the disorder in women relative to men. In Widiger and Spitzer's (1991) framework, this would represent a form of "criterion sex bias"; that is, bias inherent in the diagnostic nomenclature itself.

Recent critiques of the DSM series have argued that a particular form of "criterion sex bias" produces spurious gender differences in diagnostic prevalence rates. Specifically, several writers have suggested that sex bias on the part of clinicians and clinical researchers has influenced the construction of diagnostic criteria, causing certain disorders to be overdiagnosed in men (e.g., antisocial personality disorder) and other disorders to be overdiagnosed in women (e.g., histrionic personality disorder). In this context, critics have charged that some Axis II diagnoses reflect normal sex-role-related behaviors that have been inappropriately labeled as pathological.

Thus, Kaplan (1983) argued that the DSM-III (APA, 1980) criteria for DPD have much in common with researchers' descriptions of healthy women who happen to ascribe to the traditional female sex role. Kaplan (1983) went on to suggest that the DSM-III "singles out for scrutiny and therefore diagnosis the ways in which women express dependency but not the ways in which men express dependency" (p. 789). She pointed out that the role-related dependency of a nonworking spouse on a spouse who provides financial support (a form of dependency that has been associated with women more often than men) is regarded as symptomatic of DPD, while the types of dependent behaviors traditionally expressed by men toward women (e.g., reliance on the spouse to perform childrearing tasks and to organize and maintain the household) are ignored by the DSM-III.

Consistent with Kaplan's assertions, Landrine (1989), Sprock, Blashfield, and Smith (1990), and Rienzi and Scrams (1991) all found that mixed-sex samples of college students rated the DSM-III and DSM-III-R DPD symptom criteria as significantly more representative of traditional "feminine" behavior than of traditional "masculine" behavior.

## Gender Differences in DPD Base Rates: Fact or Artifact?

If sampling, diagnostic or criterion sex bias demonstrably influence DPD diagnoses, then observed sex differences in DPD may be artifactual. Conversely, if research suggests that these sources of bias do not affect DPD diagnoses, then we can conclude that gender differences in DPD base rates reflect genuine sex differences in the prevalence of this disorder. Thus, it is worthwhile to examine each of the possible sources of sex bias just described in the context of research on gender differences in DPD.

It does not seem likely that "sampling sex bias" is responsible for observed sex differences in the prevalence of DPD. Scrutiny of the studies listed in Table 7.1 reveals no relationship between the type of setting in which data were collected and the magnitude of sex differences in DPD base rates. Furthermore, community subjects show roughly the same magnitude of gender differences in DPD base rates as do clinical subjects (compare, for example, the prevalence of DPD in Kass et al'.s [1983] clinical and community samples). Moreover, comparable base rate differences were found in subjects from different cultures (i.e., American, Australian, Norwegian).

Along different lines, the results of two recent studies (Adler, Drake, & Teague, 1990; Loring & Powell, 1988) argue against a "diagnostic sex bias" explanation of DPD sex-difference findings. In the first of these investigations, Loring and Powell provided a number of fictitious case histories to a national sample of 290 psychiatrists and asked each psychiatrist to assign DSM-III (APA, 1980) diagnoses to the patients described in the case histories. The psychiatrists were provided with a choice of six Axis I diagnoses and six Axis II diagnoses and were permitted to assign one Axis I and one Axis II diagnosis to each patient. Patient gender was treated as an independent variable in this investigation, with some patients identified as male and some identified as female. Loring and Powell found that DPD diagnoses were assigned to 52% of the cases identified as male, but to only 39% of the cases identified as female.

Highly similar findings were subsequently reported by Adler et al. (1990), who—like Loring and Powell (1988)—assessed the effect of patient gender on diagnosticians' willingness to assign DPD diagnoses to fictitious psychiatric patients based only on case history material. A variety of diagnosticians served as subjects in Adler et al.'s study, including psychiatrists, psychiatric residents, clinical psychologists, psychiatric social workers, and psychiatric nurses. Consistent with the findings of Loring and Powell, Adler et al. (1990) found that diagnosticians did not assign DPD diagnoses more frequently to female patients than to male patients. Furthermore, Adler et al. found that male and female diagnosticians were equally likely to assign DPD diagnoses, regardless of the gender of the patient being assessed. Thus, the findings reported by Loring and Powell (1988) and Adler et al. (1990) do not support Kaplan's (1983) assertions regarding sex bias in DPD diagnoses. In fact, these findings suggest that, if anything, clinicians may actually be *less* willing to assign a DPD diagnosis to a female patient than to a male patient.

Thus, two possible explanations of the data in Table 7.1 remain. First, it is possible that women really do show higher rates of DPD than men. Second, it may be that "criterion sex bias" is inherent in the DSM-III (APA, 1980) and DSM-III-R (APA, 1987) criteria for DPD, as Kaplan's (1983) critique suggested. This question cannot be resolved through an analysis of the available data. Future researchers will need to examine this issue directly if it is to be resolved conclusively.

## NOTES

1. In fact, the proposed changes in diagnostic criteria for DPD that will appear in the DSM-IV go a long way toward correcting some of these difficulties (see APA [1991] and Hirschfeld, Shea, & Weise [1991] for detailed discussions of these proposed changes). Among the possible changes in the DSM-IV DPD symptom criteria are (1) rewording of DPD symptom 2 so that this symptom reflects the individual's inability to make major life decisions (as opposed to the more minor life decisions associated with DPD symptom 1); (2) rewording of DPD symptom 3 so that this symptom clearly reflects the dependent person's fear of losing potential caretakers; (3) extensive rewording of DPD symptom 5 so that the central component of this symptom is the individual's preoccupation with obtaining nurturance and support from others; and (4) rewording of DPD symptom 7 so that the dependent person's anxiety regarding termination of important relationships is explicitly tied to the dependent individual's desire for protection and support from others. In addition to these changes, DPD symptom 9 may be dropped from the DSM-IV because of its lack of specificity. More minor revisions may also be made in the other DPD symptom criteria. It is not clear at this point whether any or all of these proposed revisions will actually be made in the DSM-IV DPD symptom criteria. However, it is worth noting that, in general, these proposed changes will help to (1) reduce the overlap among different DPD symptoms and (2) bring the DPD symptom criteria more into line with recent empirical findings regarding the dynamics and correlates of dependent personality traits.

2. Mellsop et al. (1982) also assessed gender differences in DPD base rates. However, they did not provide enough detail regarding sample size or subject characteristics to allow their data to be compared to those obtained in other studies

of this issue. Mellsop et al. (1982) noted only that in their sample, "female patients received . . . 88% of all diagnoses of dependent personality disorder" (p. 136).

3. In this context, it is important to note that when DPD symptoms are assessed via questionnaire instead of diagnostic interview, somewhat smaller sex differences in DPD base rates are found (see Hirschfeld et al., 1991). These findings echo Yeger and Miezitis's (1985) conclusion (described in detail in Chapter 3) that observer bias may affect the degree to which dependent personality traits are attributed to men and women.

# C H A P T E R   8

# Dependency and
# Physical Disorders

Efforts to link personality traits to risk for physical illness have had a long history in psychology and psychiatry (see Alexander, French, & Pollock [1968] for a review of early studies in this area). Numerous traits have been hypothesized to place individuals at increased risk for physical illness, including anxiety, hostility, obsessiveness, aggressiveness, introversion, cynicism, and dependency. It is clear that certain of these personality traits are in fact associated with increased rates of illness and disease (Friedman & Booth-Kewley, 1987). However, in most cases causal links between the presence of particular personality traits and risk for theoretically related illnesses have not been firmly established.

As Friedman and Booth-Kewley (1987) noted, there are at least four tenable explanations for any observed personality–disease link. First, a particular personality trait might be associated with unhealthy habits and behaviors (e.g., smoking), indirectly placing an individual at risk for certain illnesses. Second, personality can affect risk for disease directly through some physiological mechanism, as in the hypothesized (but unproven) effects of "Type A" traits and behaviors on blood pressure and cardiac function. Third, an observed personality–disease link may reflect the influence of some underlying biological variable that affects—directly or indirectly—both personality and physiology (e.g., autonomic nervous system hyperresponsivity). Finally, observed personality–disease links may be due to changes in personality that follow—rather than precede—the onset of illness (e.g., increased anxiety and depression following a cancer diagnosis).

To date, most studies of the personality–disease relationship have focused on traits such as cynicism, aggressiveness, and hostility. However, during the past 40 years there have also been a number of investigations examining possible links between dependency and risk for physical illness. In this chapter I review empirical evidence regarding the dependency–

disease relationship. First, I discuss the historical roots of present-day research on the dependency–disease link. Next, I review the empirical literature on dependency as a risk factor for physical illness. Finally, I discuss studies that allow me to formulate some tentative hypotheses regarding the causal links between dependent personality traits and risk for illness and disease.

## THE DEPENDENCY–DISEASE LINK: HISTORICAL ROOTS

The hypothesis that exaggerated or unexpressed dependency needs would place an individual at increased risk for physical illness is rooted in at least three sources. First and foremost, Alexander's (1950) seminal work on the psychodynamics of psychosomatic disorders postulated that when the expression of dependency needs or aggressive impulses was blocked, an individual was put at risk for a variety of physical illnesses. Alexander hypothesized that unexpressed dependency needs would result in persistent stimulation of the parasympathetic nervous system, thereby increasing the likelihood that an individual would develop disorders such as ulcers, colitis, and asthma. Conversely, Alexander hypothesized that unexpressed aggressive impulses would result in chronic sympathetic nervous system arousal and ultimately in increased risk for hypertension, heart disease, and other illnesses.

It is noteworthy that Alexander (1950; Alexander et al., 1968) not only specified the neurological correlates of various psychosomatic illnesses, but futhermore offered specific hypotheses regarding which illnesses would result from particular psychodynamic conflicts. In describing the findings that resulted from their initial studies in this area, Alexander et al. (1968) noted:

> [T]he psychological situation in which the patient found himself at the onset of his physical symptoms—which we call the *onset situation*—consisted precisely in the activation of the characteristic psychodynamic conflict pattern that had been present from childhood on. . . . Thus, in ulcer patients it makes physiological sense that frustrated dependent, help-seeking desires should have a specific correlation to stomach activity, the connecting link being the association between the wish to be loved and helped and the wish to be fed. (p. 7)

When Alexander et al. (1968) conducted a large-scale investigation of the personality–disease relationship in a mixed-sex sample of adult medical patients, their hypotheses regarding the link between dependency and ulcers were generally confirmed: Alexander et al. were able to distinguish ulcer patients from other medical patients at better-than-chance level using only information related to the patients' attitudes toward—and behavior regarding—dependency. Moreover, the percentage of correct diagnoses made by Alexander et al. based on interview-derived ratings of the patients' "psychodynamic conflicts" (34%) actually exceeded the percentage of correct diagnoses made by physicians who based their conclusions only on the patients' physical symptoms (31%). Similar findings were obtained for a variety of other disorders (e.g., asthma, neurodermatitis, hypertension, colitis).

Around the same time that Alexander (1950) published his initial work on the personality–disease relationship, Reusch (1948) speculated that the presence of an "infantile personality" was the core problem in many—if not most—forms of psychosomatic illness. The "infantile personality" of which Reusch spoke was in fact a precursor of what eventually became the passive–dependent personality in the DSM-I (APA, 1952) and DSM-II (APA, 1968). Reusch's "infantile personality" also had much in common with DPD as it is described in the DSM-III (APA, 1980) and DSM-III-R (APA, 1987), and with recent clinical descriptions of dependent individuals (e.g., Birtchnell, 1988a; Millon, 1981; Turkat & Carlson, 1984). A brief quotation from Reusch's work illustrates these parallels. Reusch (1948) speculated that the "infantile" person cannot "form clear-cut and consistent proprioceptive cues which would enable the individual to proceed on his own. . . . Instead, he relies upon cues received from others, which necessitates permanent guidance and support by others" (p. 138).

Unlike Alexander (1950), Reusch (1948) did not describe specific personality–disease links in his discussion of psychosomatic illness. Instead, Reusch (1948) simply conjectured in general terms that "breakdown of immature personalities occurs when reliance upon the external security system is impossible, when there is no model to be copied, when personalized rewards in terms of affection are unobtainable, or when independent action is necessary" (p. 139). Reusch's failure to outline specific dependency–disease links caused his work to be somewhat less influential than Alexander's work during the 1950s and 1960s. Nonetheless, Reusch's ideas stimulated a number of investigations in this area and continue to be widely cited by researchers examining the personality–disease link (see Ammon, 1979; Greenberg & Bornstein, 1988a; Greenberg & Dattore, 1981; Vaillant, 1978).

Finally, human and animal studies conducted during the 1960s and 1970s suggested that chronic helplessness and hopelessness—either characterological or experimentally induced—were associated with increased risk for a variety of physical illnesses, including heart disease and cancer (see Temoshok [1987] for a review of these experiments). Because helplessness has long been regarded by researchers as a central feature of the dependent personality (see Fisher & Greenberg, 1985; Masling, 1986; Millon, 1981), these studies provided indirect evidence supporting the hypothesis that dependency might predispose individuals to the development of physical illness.

## THE DEPENDENCY–DISEASE LINK: EMPIRICAL EVIDENCE

Researchers have examined possible relationships between dependency and a variety of physical disorders (e.g., ulcers, colitis, diabetes, asthma, epilepsy, arthritis, tuberculosis, cancer, heart disease). In most of these investigations, dependency was found to be associated with elevated rates of illness (see Masling & Schwartz [1979] for a detailed discussion of these findings). However, because the vast majority of studies in this area used correlational designs, it is impossible to draw strong conclusions regarding causal relationships among the variables assessed in these investigations.

Studies of the dependency–asthma relationship are a case in point. Although several studies found that asthmatic subjects obtained significantly higher dependency scores than did nonasthmatic controls (e.g., Harris, 1956; Khampalikit, 1983; Langveld, 1954; Meijer, 1981; Williams, 1975), it is impossible to tell from these data whether dependency preceded or followed the onset of asthmatic illness. This is particularly problematic because research suggests that the onset of serious physical illness is often followed by an increase in dependent feelings and behaviors, even in individuals who earlier had shown no signs of exaggerated dependency needs (Greenberg & Bornstein, 1988a; Saviola, 1981; Viederman, 1974). Furthermore, reinforcement of passive, "sick" behavior by friends and caretakers can produce an increase in self-reports of symptoms of a preexisting physical disorder as well as an increase in dependent, help-seeking behaviors (Henderson, 1974; Hoare, 1984; Stores & Piran, 1978). Moreover, as discussed in Chapter 7, the experience of being hospitalized and treated for physical or psychological illness can—in and of itself—produce increases in dependent behavior.

Although dependency has been linked to a wide variety of physical illnesses in isolated, unreplicated studies, the relationship between dependency and two physical disorders—ulcers and cancer—has been studied more extensively via well-designed correlational and longitudinal investigations. Stronger conclusions regarding the dependency–disease link can be drawn from the results of these studies.

Most studies of the dependency–ulcers relationship have found that ulcer patients obtain significantly higher dependency scores (assessed via a variety of measures including the ROD scale, 16PF, MMPI Dy scale, and Blacky test) than do matched groups of nonulcer control patients (Alexander et al., 1968; Magni, Rizzardo, & DiMario, 1984; Magni, Salmi, &

Paterlini, 1982; McIntosh, Nasiry, & Frysman, 1983; Rothstein & Cohen, 1958; Sharma & Rao, 1974; Spiesman & Singer, 1961; Streitfeld, 1954; Weiss & Emmerich, 1962; Weiss & Masling, 1970; Wolowitz, 1967; Wolowitz & Wagonfeld, 1968). There have been more than a dozen empirical studies of the dependency–ulcers relationship conducted to date, and only three of these investigations (i.e., Berger, 1959; Kanter & Hazelton, 1964; Pollie, 1964) have failed to find a dependency–ulcers link.

Furthermore, two studies suggest a possible causal relationship between dependent personality traits and the later development of ulcers. In an early investigation, Weiner, Thaler, Reiser, and Mirsky (1957) found higher levels of baseline (i.e., resting state) pepsinogen secretion in dependent than nondependent male army draftees. Moreover, those draftees with higher resting state pepsinogen secretion rates subsequently showed higher rates of duodenal ulcers than did draftees with lower resting state pepsinogen secretion rates. Similar results were recently obtained by Magni, DiMario, Rizzardo, Pulin, and Naccarato (1986). In this study, dependency (assessed via the 16PF) predicted resting state pepsinogen secretion rates (as well as ulcer rates) in a mixed-sex sample of 79 Italian medical patients.

The results of Weiner et al.'s (1957) and Magni et al.'s (1986) investigations suggest that higher baseline anxiety or autonomic arousal levels in dependent than nondependent individuals might play a role in the dependency–ulcers link. Specifically, higher anxiety or arousal levels might cause dependent persons to secrete greater amounts of pepsinogen than do nondependent persons, ultimately leading to higher ulcer rates in dependent individuals. However, dependent individuals do not show higher rates of generalized anxiety disorder than nondependent individuals (Alnaes & Torgerson, 1988b; Reich et al., 1987), nor do they show higher baseline levels of autonomic arousal than nondependent individuals (Masling et al., 1981; Masling, Bornstein, Poynton, Reed, & Katkin, 1991). Thus, the hypothesis of a "generalized anxiety" link between dependency and ulcers is not supported by relevant empirical findings.

The results of two quasi-experimental studies suggest that a specific form of anxiety—that is, anxiety regarding interpersonal conflict and the disruption of interpersonal relationships—may mediate the dependency–ulcers link. Luborsky and Auerbach (1969) utilized data from verbatim recordings of psychotherapy sessions to compare the verbalizations of a 25-year-old male ulcer patient that occurred (1) immediately before an exacerbation of stomach symptoms versus (2) before nonpain periods. Periods of stomach pain were significantly more likely than nonpain periods to be preceded by themes of helplessness and interpersonal conflict. A subsequent reanalysis of these data by Spence (1970) further indicated that words associated with dependency occurred significantly more often before pain periods than before nonpain periods.

Results from studies of the dependency–cancer relationship parallel the results obtained in studies of the dependency–ulcers relationship (see Greenberg & Bornstein [1988a] for a detailed description of these findings). Early work in this area confirmed the existence of dependency–cancer link in both men (Greene, 1954; LeShan & Worthington, 1956) and women (Greene, Young, & Swisher, 1956; Reznikoff, 1955). Furthermore, these studies indicated that dependency predicted the development of a variety of carcinomas, including breast cancer, prostate cancer, colon cancer, and leukemia. These initial results were replicated and extended by Bahnson and Bahnson (1964a, 1964b, 1966), who also found dependency to predict the development of a variety of cancers.

Two particularly well-designed longitudinal studies (Greenberg & Dattore, 1981; Vaillant, 1978) not only suggest that dependency is a risk factor for ulcers and cancer, but further indicate that dependency predisposes an individual to a variety of physical disorders. Greenberg and Dattore compared the MMPI Dy scores of male VA patients who later developed cancer ($n = 58$) or one of three other physical disorders (i.e., benign tumors, hypertension, or gastrointestinal ulcers) ($n = 42$) to the Dy scores of a control group of men who remained disease-free for the 10-year period following the initial dependency screening ($n = 37$). Greenberg and Dattore (1981) found that men who subsequently developed any of the physical disorders that were assessed in this study showed significantly higher initial dependency scores than did men who remained disease-free for the duration of the investigation. Moreover, Greenberg and Dattore found that several other dependency-related MMPI scaled (i.e., "dependency urge," "dependency in action," "repression of dependency," and "dependency frustration") (see Finney [1965, 1966] for detailed descriptions of these scales) also predicted the subsequent onset of various physical disorders in members of their subject sample.

Consistent with the findings of Greenberg and Dattore, Vaillant (1978) found that dependency was a "nonspecific" risk factor for subsequent physical illness in nonclinical (i.e., college student) subjects. In Vaillant's investigation, level of dependency assessed during late adolescence predicted the development of ulcers, hypertension, colitis, allergies, and musculoskeletal problems in a sample of male college graduates followed over a 30-year period (cancer rates were not assessed in Vaillant's study). Vaillant found that dependency predicted the development of a variety of physical problems but did not predict the form that illness would take.

It is informative to compare the magnitude of the dependency–disease relationships obtained by Greenberg and Dattore (1981) and Vaillant (1978) with the magnitude of the relationships between various personality traits and risk for physical illness that were reported by Friedman and Booth-Kewley (1987) in their meta-analytic review of research on the "disease-prone personality." Friedman and Booth-Kewley examined research assessing the relationship of several personality dimensions (i.e., anxiety, depression, anger, hostility, aggression, introversion) to risk for several physical illnesses (i.e., heart disease, asthma, ulcers, arthritis, migraine headaches). Correlations between level of a given personality trait and risk for disease ranged from $-.01$ (for anger and hostility as predictors of risk for ulcers and headaches) to .32 (for anxiety as a predictor of asthma) in Friedman and Booth-Kewley's meta-analysis.

By employing the procedures recommended by Rosenthal (1984), it was possible to derive overall personality–disease correlations (using the effect size estimate $r$) from the information provided by Friedman and Booth-Kewley (1987). The personality dimension that best predicted risk for physical illness (in general) in Friedman and Booth-Kewley's meta-analysis was anxiety, wherein a mean correlation of .20 between level of anxiety and risk for disease was found. The personality dimension that was the worst predictor of physical illness was introversion ($r = .04$). Other personality dimensions also produced modest (albeit statistically significant) personality–disease correlations (i.e., depression, $r = .15$; anger/hostility, $r = .11$; anger/hostility/aggression, $r = .10$). Overall, the mean personality–disease correlation in Friedman and Booth-Kewley's (1987) meta-analysis was .10.

In contrast, Vaillant (1978) found a correlation of .35 between level of dependency assessed at age 20 and global physical illness ratings obtained at age 50. The magnitude of the dependency–disease relationship in Greenberg and Dattore's and Vaillant's (1981) longitudinal sample was .19. Thus, comparison of Greenberg and Dattore's and Vaillant's (1978) findings with those of Friedman and Booth-Kewley (1987) indicates that level of dependency is at least as strong a predictor of risk for physical illness as are other theoretically related personality traits. In fact, dependency may actually be a somewhat better predictor of risk for disease than are these other traits. The fact that the magnitude of the dependency–disease link in Greenberg and Dattore's and Vaillant's longitudinal studies exceeded the magnitude of the personality–disease relationship obtained by Friedman and Booth-Kewley is particularly noteworthy because Friedman and Booth-Kewley included both correlational and longitudinal data in their meta-analysis (which would tend to inflate any observed dependency–disease correlations), while Greenberg and Dattore and Vaillant utilized only longitudinal data in their investigations.

## SOME POSSIBLE MECHANISMS UNDERLYING THE DEPENDENCY–DISEASE RELATIONSHIP

Although it is clear that dependency is a risk factor for physical illness, the mechanism by which dependency increases an individual's risk for physical disorders remains unknown. Several variables have been hypothesized to mediate the dependency–disease link. For example, Vaillant (1978, 1983) suggested that higher rates of tobacco and alcohol use among dependent individuals might increase their risk for a variety of physical disorders. Vaillant's hypotheses is a variant of the "unhealthy habits and behaviors" personality–disease link described by Friedman and Booth-Kewley (1987). The studies discussed in Chapter 6 which demonstrated that dependency is indeed associated with high levels of alcohol and tobacco use are consistent with Vaillant's hypothesis.

Bornstein et al. (1990) proposed a somewhat different mechanism to account for the dependency–disease relationship, suggesting that the defensive style of the dependent person might increase her risk for certain illnesses. Bornstein et al.'s hypothesis is essentially a variant of the "direct influence" personality–disease link described by Friedman and Booth-Kewley (1987). Numerous studies have demonstrated that the defensive style that Bornstein et al. (1990) and Levit (1991) found to be associated with dependency (i.e., a defensive style characterized by inward-directed rather than outwardly expressed anger) is also associated with increased risk for a variety of physical disorders (see Chesney & Rosenman, 1985; Ihilevich & Gleser, 1986; Temoshok, 1987). These studies offer indirect support for Bornstein et al.'s suggestions in this area.

Along different lines, Greenberg and Bornstein (1988a) hypothesized that the link between dependency and the subsequent development of disease may lie in the dependent person's exaggerated response to the termination (or perceived threat of termination) of important interpersonal relationships. Berscheid and Fei (1977), Buunk (1982, 1983) and others have shown that dependency is associated with increased anxiety, jealousy, and insecurity in close interpersonal relationships. Thus, Greenberg and Bornstein (1988a) suggested that when important relationships end or are threatened, "early feelings of helplessness and isolation re-emerge [in the dependent person] . . . a lifetime of excessive reliance on external expressions of love and reassurance results in a traumatic reaction when the eventual loss, or threat of loss, of the love object takes place" (p. 128). In other words, Greenberg and Bornstein hypothesized that dependency acts as a diathesis that—when coupled with events in the environment that activate feelings of dependency and helplessness—places an individual at risk for a variety of physical illnesses.

Although Greenberg and Bornstein's (1988a) hypothesis regarding the possible role of "relationship anxiety" in mediating the dependency–disease link has not been tested directly, several sets of findings offer indirect support for this hypothesis. For example, Luborsky and Auerbach's (1969) findings (described earlier) regarding the content of verbalizations that preceded the exacerbation of stomach ulcer symptoms in a male psychotherapy patient are consistent with Greenberg and Bornstein's "relationship anxiety" hypothesis (see also Alexander et al., 1968; Spence, 1970).

Additional indirect support for Greenberg and Bornstein's (1988a) hypothesis comes from the work of Bahnson and Bahnson (1964a, 1964b, 1966), who found that the interpersonal relationships of dependent individuals who later developed cancer were characterized by insecurity, "clinging dependency," jealousy, and possessiveness on the part of the dependent person. Moreover, in a prospective study, Thomas and Duszynski (1974) found that medical students who reported interpersonal isolation and feelings of loneliness were more likely to develop a variety of physical disorders than were members of a matched control group of students who did not report problems in these areas. Similarly, Graves, Mead, and Pearson (1986) found that medical students with problematic or impoverished interpersonal relationships were at increased risk for heart disease.

Along slightly different lines, several investigations have examined possible links between the disruption of important interpersonal relationships and mortality and illness rates. In this context, Bahnson (1975), Schmale (1958), Engel (1967), and Paffanbarger, Wolf, Notkin, and Thorne (1966) all found that early disruption of parental relationships predicted the subsequent development of a variety of physical disorders. Paffanbarger et al.'s (1966) results are typical of those obtained in this area. They reported that the early death of either parent was associated with a 50–75% increase in the incidence of heart disease in nonclinical (i.e., college student) subjects. Paffanbarger et al.'s results parallel Spitz's (1965) well-known finding that disruption of the maternal relationship during the first few years of life leads to increased risk for a variety of physical illnesses, and to increases in mortality rates as well (see Bowlby, 1953; Stendler, 1954).

Unfortunately, no studies have examined directly the interaction of dependency and interpersonal stress as risk factors for physical illness. Clearly, dependency and interpersonal stress both predict illness and disease rates, even in nonclinical subjects. Whether dependency and interpersonal stress interact to further increase an individual's risk for physical illness—as Greenberg and Bornstein (1988a) hypothesized—is an empirical issue that has not yet been addressed conclusively.

The question remains: What is the physiological link between "relationship anxiety" and risk for physical illness? We can only speculate at this point. Perhaps the dependent individual's "relationship anxiety" increases his or her risk for a variety of diseases by diminishing immune system response. The deleterious effects of chronic stress on immunocompetence have been documented on a number of occasions (see, e.g., Jemmot & Locke, 1984; Levine, Wiener, & Coe, 1989). Most recently, the negative effects of chronic stress on immune system function were confirmed in an extensive review of the empirical literature on this topic by O'Leary (1990).

O'Leary not only examined the empirical literature demonstrating the existence of a stress–immune function link and assessed the role of interpersonal stress in inhibiting immune function, she also provided evidence that certain personality traits (e.g., inhibited power motivation, external locus of control) may mediate the stress–immune function relationship.

Unfortunately, the possible role of dependency as a risk factor for stress-based immune system deficiencies was not discussed by O'Leary (1990). Nonetheless, the hypothesis that stress-based immune system deficiencies may mediate the dependency–disease link is indirectly supported by a series of studies conducted by Kiecolt-Glaser, Pennebaker, and their colleagues (e.g., Kiecolt-Glaser et al., 1987; Pennebaker & Beall, 1986; Pennebaker, Kiecolt-Glaser, & Glaser, 1988). In these investigations, actual and perceived disruptions of significant interpersonal relationships were found to result in diminished immunocompetence, both in normal subjects and in members of clinical (i.e., medical or psychiatric) populations. Similarly, Bartrop, Luckhurst, Lazarus, Kiloh, and Penny (1977) found that bereavement-related stress produced long-term inhibition of immune system function in a mixed-sex sample of 26 recently widowed adults.

Furthermore, paralleling the findings obtained by Hammen et al. (1985, 1989a, 1989b) regarding dependency, interpersonal stress, and risk for depression (see Chapter 6 for a detailed description of these studies), Kiecolt-Glaser, Pennebaker, and their colleagues found that high levels of interpersonal stressors were associated with increased rates of physical illness in both normal and clinical subjects (see, e.g., Kiecolt-Glaser et al., 1987; Pennebaker et al., 1988). Although these researchers did not assess dependency as a possible mediating variable in the interpersonal stress–immune function link (cf. Bartrop et al., 1977), their results nonetheless suggest that dependent individuals' concern with obtaining and maintaining nurturant, supportive interpersonal relationships might indirectly place them at increased risk for diseases mediated by immune system response.

Thus, although the mechanism by which dependency increases a person's risk for physical disorders remains open to question, it seems likely that the dependency–disease link represents an instance in which personality exerts a "direct influence" on risk for disease (Friedman & Booth-Kewley, 1987), most likely by diminishing immune system response. In any case, in one important respect findings regarding the dependency–disease link are straightforward and unambiguous: In contrast to findings form prospective and experimental studies of the dependency–psychopathology relationship, where different results were obtained for different areas of psychopathology, prospective studies of the dependency–disease relationship converge to indicate that dependency is a generalized risk factor for a wide variety of physical illnesses.

# *Dependency and Patienthood*

Investigations of dependency and various patient-related behaviors make explicit the fact that the relationship between a patient and his or her doctor is, first and foremost, characterized by social exchange (even if most of that social exchange happens to center around the patient's physical or psychological symptoms). Thus, research examining the impact of dependency on patient-related behaviors provides a unique opportunity to link studies assessing the interpersonal correlates of dependency with studies of dependency and physical or psychological disorders. With this in mind, one would expect to find parallels between the behavior exhibited by dependent persons in social settings and that exhibited by dependent persons in clinical settings.

For example, in light of the findings discussed in Chapter 4 regarding dependent persons' cooperative, compliant behavior toward figures of authority, it seems likely that dependency will be an important determinant of the behavior exhibited by patients in clinical settings, where figures of authority (e.g., physicians, therapists) abound. Moreover, as discussed in Chapter 8, the onset of an episode of illness tends to produce increases in dependent behavior even in persons who do not ordinarily show exaggerated dependency needs. Thus, not only would one expect to find a general increase in the amount of dependent behavior exhibited by individuals upon entering the clinical setting, but one would also expect that much of this behavior will be directed toward physicians, nurses, psychologists, and other individuals who simultaneously represent pseudo-parental authority figures and potential caretakers.

In fact, based on the findings discussed in Chapter 4 regarding the behavior of dependent persons in social settings, it is possible to generate several specific, testable predictions regarding the behavior of dependent individuals in clinical settings. First, given the help-seeking style of the dependent person, dependent individuals should be more likely than nondependent individuals to seek medical or psychological help when symptoms appear. Similarly, dependent persons in a psychiatric setting should show a help-seeking response set on psychological tests. Furthermore, the dependent person should be reluctant to terminate a medical or psychotherapeutic relationship because terminating these relationships involves losing a powerful caretaker (the physician or therapist), which the dependent person will be reluctant to do.

Second, research on suggestibility, yielding, and compliance suggests that dependent individuals are highly motivated to please figures of authority. If compliant, cooperative behavior is exhibited by dependent individuals in social and academic settings, dependency should be associated with similar kinds of behaviors in medical settings, perhaps to an even greater degree. Thus, dependency should be associated with compliance with medical and psychological treatment regimens.

Third, research on interpersonal sensitivity has demonstrated that dependent persons are sensitive to social cues and make accurate inferences regarding the attitudes and beliefs of acquaintances, roommates, and teachers. It is likely that dependent persons will be highly motivated to discover the attitudes and beliefs of an important caretaking figure such as a physician or psychologist. Thus, dependent persons should be more accurate than nondependent persons in making inferences regarding the attitudes and beliefs of doctors and therapists.

Anecdotal evidence from case studies of dependent psychiatric and medical patients is consistent with each of the hypotheses just described (see, e.g., Barry et al., 1965; Berry, 1986; Blatt, 1974; Emery & Lesher, 1982; Handler, 1989; Hopkins, 1986; Lomas, 1965; Lower, 1967; Overholser, 1987; Pakes, 1975; Parens & Saul, 1971; Snyder, 1963; Turkat & Carlson, 1984). The descriptions of dependent persons in these case studies echo clearly many of the empirical findings regarding the dependent personality that have been discussed thus far. Turkat and Carlson's description of a 48-year-old female psychotherapy patient illustrates the general tone and content of the clinical descriptions of dependent patients that are contained in most of these case reports. Turkat and Carlson (1984) noted:

> [The patient] reported numerous decision-making situations which provoked anxiety and attempts to seek reassurance. . . . Further, she reported feeling anxious when the availability of her husband's reassurance was denied. . . . Assessment of early upbringing revealed the patient's lack of independent decision-making . . . she reported that her father "always told me what to do" and that "he did not permit me to be independent at all" . . . . The patient described her upbringing as one in which her parents "mapped out what I was to do and not to do" . . . . . During school years, she always wanted to be part of the "group," but felt uncomfortable because no one would explicitly point out that she did in fact fit in. . . . When the patient went to college, she studied

nursing because "a lot of people my age went into nursing" .... The patient's first job as a nurse went smoothly because she had readily available supervisors. Unfortunately, her second position did not fare well. Apparently, Mrs. S had trouble adjusting because she did not have supportive supervisors. . . . She was greatly attracted to her husband because he was "very forceful" and an "independent decision-maker." (pp. 156–157)

Turkat and Carlson's (1984) clinical description captures many of the important empirical results obtained in studies of dependency and the dependent personality, including findings regarding the role of parental authoritarianism in the etiology of adult dependency (Chapter 3), as well as findings regarding the compliant, help-seeking behaviors of the dependent person in social and academic settings (Chapter 4). Other case studies and clinical descriptions of dependent psychiatric patients are also consistent with many of the empirical findings described in earlier chapters (see, e.g., Hopkins, 1986; Lomas, 1965; Parens & Saul, 1971).

In addition to presenting case material illustrating the personality dynamics of dependent individuals, several writers have discussed the kinds of difficulties that are frequently encountered in working with dependent psychiatric and medical patients. For example, Emery and Lesher (1982) suggested that dependent psychotherapy patients differ from nondependent patients on 12 primary dimensions. Specifically, Emery and Lesher argued that during psychotherapy, dependent patients tend to (1) overdisclose intimate details of their personal lives; (2) become emotionally labile when frustrated; (3) arrive early for sessions; (4) willingly comply with the therapist's instructions and "homework" assignments; (5) present numerous major and minor problems to the therapist; (6) attempt to shift responsibility for solving these problems to the therapist; (7) try to extend the length of psychotherapy sessions; (8) resist termination; (9) express doubts regarding their ability to function independently; (10) make numerous overt requests for advice and reassurance; (11) assume a passive, helpless stance during psychotherapy; and (12) overreact to minor personal crises.

Two aspects of Emery and Lesher's (1982) clinical material are particularly noteworthy in the present context. First, these writers' observations parallel those of Balint (1964) and others (e.g., Dollard & Miller, 1950), who suggested that dependency is associated with both positive and negative treatment-related behaviors (see Chapter 1 for a detailed discussion of earlier views regarding the treatment-related behaviors of dependent psychiatric and medical patients). Second, Emery and Lesher's observations suggest that patient dependency may play an important role in transference and countertransference dynamics (see, e.g., behaviors 1, 2, 6, 7, 10, and 11, listed above). Insofar as dependency is associated with patient cooperativeness and/or resistance, dependency will have a significant impact on the therapist–patient relationship and on the course and outcome of psychotherapy.

Of course, while case material such as that described by Turkat and Carlson (1984) and Emery and Lesher (1982) is interesting (and potentially heuristic), it is not useful in testing rigorously hypotheses regarding the relationship of dependency to various patient-related behaviors. Fortunately, there have been a number of empirical studies that address these hypotheses directly. In the following sections, I discuss the relationship of dependency to (1) help-seeking behavior in clinical settings; (2) compliance with treatment regimens; and (3) perceptions of the psychotherapist and the psychotherapeutic process.

## DEPENDENCY AND HELP SEEKING IN CLINICAL SETTINGS

Studies of dependency and help seeking in clinical settings can be divided into three domains. First, a number of researchers have assessed the relationship between dependency and treatment delay in medical patients. Second, several researchers have examined the relationship between dependency and help-seeking behavior in inpatient and outpatient psychological treatment. Third, a few researchers have investigated the relationship between patient dependency and length of treatment for medical and psychological disorders.

### Dependency and Treatment Delay

A number of studies have-found that dependency predicts delay in seeking treatment when physical symptoms appear (Brown & Rawlinson, 1975; Fisher, 1967; Geersten & Gray, 1970; Greenberg & Fisher, 1977; Hammerschlag, Fisher, DeCosse, & Kaplan, 1964; Phillips, 1965; Stamler & Palmer, 1971; Zeldow & Greenberg, 1979, 1980). In each of these investigations, high dependency scores were associated with shorter delay in seeking treatment following symptom onset. Unfortunately, no studies have examined the dependency–treatment delay relationship for psychological symptoms. Nonetheless, the dependency–treatment delay relationship has been found for numerous medical disorders, including heart disease (Brown & Rawlinson, 1975), breast cancer (Hammerschlag et al., 1964), and other forms of cancer (see Fisher, 1967). In addition, the dependency–treatment delay relationship is obtained regardless of whether projective (Fisher, 1967) or self-report measures of dependency (Greenberg & Fisher, 1977) are used. Finally, the dependency–treatment delay relationship is found in both children (Stamler & Palmer, 1971) and adults (Zeldow & Greenberg, 1979, 1980).

Greenberg and Fisher's (1977) findings illustrate the pattern of results typically obtained in studies in this area, and further suggest that the dependency–treatment delay relationship holds for a wide variety of physical symptoms. Greenberg and Fisher examined the correlations between self-reports of interpersonal dependency and subjects' estimates of the amount of time (in days) that they believed they would delay before seeking treatment following the onset of various types of physical symptoms. Subjects in this study were 28 adult women who were not currently undergoing treatment for medical or psychiatric disorders.

The central findings of Greenberg and Fisher's (1977) investigation are summarized in Table 9.1. As this table shows, the dependency–treatment delay relationship is fairly consistent across symptom type. Dependency-delay correlations ranged from a low of −.30 (for upper body symptoms) to a high of −.56 (for symptoms associated with significant pain or discomfort). The mean dependency–delay correlation for the eight classes of symptoms listed in Table 9.1 was −.40. Highly similar findings were obtained by Stamler and Palmer (1971), who reported a correlation of −.30 between projective dependency scores and chart-derived indices of treatment delay in a mixed-sex sample of elementary school children.

These findings raise an important question: What accounts for the inverse relationship between dependency and treatment delay? One possibility is that dependent persons are more willing than nondependent persons to enter into a doctor–patient relationship, wherein they submit to the advice and direction of an omniscient, omnipotent caretaker (see Juni & Fischer [1983] for a detailed discussion of this hypothesis). If this is the case, then it is likely that dependent persons have different attitudes than do

TABLE 9.1. Correlations between Dependency Scores and Estimates of Treatment Delay in Greenberg and Fisher's Study

| Type of symptom | Dependency–delay correlation |
|---|---|
| Exterior | −.50** |
| Interior | −.33* |
| Upper body | −.30 |
| Lower body | −.49** |
| Painful | −.56** |
| Nonpainful | −.31 |
| Physical | −.45** |
| Psychiatric | −.49** |

*Note. n* of subjects included in this table = 28.
*$p < .05$. **$p < .01$.
Adapted from Greenberg and Fisher (1977, Table 1). © 1977 by Pergamon Press. Adapted by permission of the publisher.

nondependent persons regarding medical treatment. Specifically, dependent persons should have more positive attitudes than do nondependent persons regarding physicians and hospitals. Two sets of findings address this question.

First, Greenberg and Fisher (1977) found that dependent women gave more positive descriptions than did nondependent women of (1) a "typical" physician and (2) a "typical" hospital stay. The dependent women in Greenberg and Fisher's study viewed the typical physician as warmer and more pleasant than did the nondependent women, and perceived the typical hospital stay as more pleasant. Furthermore, the dependent women in this study reported that their most recent interactions with physicians were generally positive, while nondependent women described recent interactions with physicians in more negative terms. These findings are consistent with the hypothesis that dependent persons have more positive attitudes than do nondependent persons regarding physicians and hospitals. Needless to say, if physicians and hospitals are perceived in a positive way by the dependent person, the dependent individual will be more likely than the nondependent individual to utilize medical and psychological services.

A study by Parker and Lipscombe (1980) suggests that the origin of dependent persons' positive attitudes toward physicians and hospitals may lie in early learning and socialization experiences within the family. Parker and Lipscombe examined the relationship between DEQ dependency scores and retrospective reports of parents' reactions to childhood illness in a mixed-sex sample of adult medical patients. A number of interesting findings were obtained in this investigation, but three results in particular are noteworthy in the present context. The parents of dependent patients were more likely than the parents of nondependent patients to (1) take an episode of childhood illness seriously; (2) show sympathy and concern regarding the illness; and (3) seek the advice of a physician when the child became ill. Thus, dependent persons' positive attitudes toward physicians and medical treatment appear to be an indirect result of their parents' positive attitudes in these areas. Moreover, the dependent person's tendency to seek treatment relatively soon after symptom onset may reflect his parents' tendency to seek the advice of a physician when their child became ill.

Along different lines, several studies have found that dependent women are more likely than nondependent women to view somatic problems as having a medical rather than a psychological cause (see Greenberg & Fisher, 1977; Phillips, 1965; Zeldow & Greenberg, 1979, 1980). In fact, studies by Bornstein et al. (1988b), Fisher and Fisher (1975), and Strack, Lorr, Campbell, and Lamnin (1992) indicate that dependency is associated with a generalized tendency to report somatic symptoms even when healthy. Apparently, dependent individuals are preoccupied with concerns regarding physical illness and have a tendency to develop somatic symptoms when under stress (see Fisher [1970] for a detailed discussion of this issue). These findings may help to explain why dependent persons seek treatment relatively quickly following symptom onset: To the extent that somatic symptoms are viewed as reflecting physical illness, an individual will be more likely to consult a physician regarding the symptoms.

Consistent with the findings of Strack et al. (1992) and others, Morrison, Bushell, Hanson, Fentiman, and Holdridge-Crane (1977) found that dependent psychiatric outpatients were more likely than nondependent outpatients to conceptualize mental illness in medical (rather than psychosocial) terms. Agoustinos (1986) obtained virtually identical results in a mixed-sex sample of psychiatric inpatients. Although Wehler (1979) reported a nonsignificant relationship between dependency and medical orientation toward mental illness in a sample of psychiatric inpatients, his results were in the predicted direction: While Morrison et al. (1977) obtained a correlation of .60 between dependency and an index of medical orientation in members of their outpatient sample, and Agoustinos obtained a correlation of .50 between these two variables in her inpatient subjects, Wehler reported a correlation of .15 between dependency and medical orientation scores in his sample of inpatients.

## Dependency and Help Seeking

Not surprisingly, when dependent individuals seek treatment for psychological problems, research suggests that they adopt a help-seeking attitude. Two different paradigms have been used to examine this issue. In one paradigm, help seeking is assessed from MMPI validity scale scores. Using this approach, O'Neill and Bornstein (1990) derived an index of "help-seeking response set" from the MMPI validity scales (i.e., $F - K$) see Gough, 1950) of a mixed-sex sample of 101 voluntary psychiatric inpatients who completed the MMPI as part of a standard psychological testing battery routinely administered to patients upon admission to the psychiatric unit. ROD scores were calculated from Rorschach protocols that had been administered as part of the same psychological testing battery. O'Neill and Bornstein found that, as predicted, dependency was associated with help-seeking response set on the MMPI (i.e., high $F$ and low $K$ score), in both men and women. In fact, the correlation between ROD scores and $F - K$ scores was quite substantial ($r = .52$) in O'Neill and Bornstein's study.

A very different approach to investigating the dependency–help-seeking relationship was used by Lorr and McNair (1964b). In this study, 150 male outpatients undergoing treatment for a variety of psychological disorders were rated by their primary therapists for the degree to which they exhibited each of 32 patient-related behaviors during psychotherapy sessions. Ratings were made for each patient following the fourth therapy session. Lorr and McNair then examined the correlation between these therapist-derived ratings and measures of each patient's overall level of dependency.

The central findings of Lorr and McNair's (1964b) investigation are summarized in Table 9.2, which lists the 10 behavior descriptors that showed the strongest correlations with patients' overall dependency scores. As this table shows, dependent psychiatric patients are viewed by their therapists as exhibiting a wide range of compliant, help-seeking behaviors during therapy. In fact, the three behavior descriptors that were most strongly associated with overall level of dependency in Lorr and McNair's investigation clearly reflect a help-seeking stance on the part of the patient. Moreover, 6 of the 10 items in Table 9.2 (i.e., items 1, 2, 3, 4, 5, and 10) are associated with passivity, help seeking, and compliance.

**TABLE 9.2. The 10 Patient-Related Behaviors Most Strongly Correlated with Psychiatric Patients' Overall Dependency Scores in Lorr and McNair's Study**

| Patient-related behavior | Correlation with overall dependency score |
|---|---|
| 1. Relies on you for support or reassurance | .72 |
| 2. Seeks or requests direct advice and guidance | .68 |
| 3. Submissively and passively solicits help | .64 |
| 4. Uses "Dr." and "Sir" and other means of showing subordination and respect | .40 |
| 5. Tries to tease opinions, interpretations, or evalutions from you | .38 |
| 6. Emphasizes his problems, unacceptable feelings, motives, or traits | .28 |
| 7. Shows close and positive rapport | .28 |
| 8. Openly expresses resentment and hostility toward you | .28 |
| 9. Fails to allow your remarks and comments to register or "sink in" | .27 |
| 10. Talks about his need for medical help, medication, or treatment of his physical symptoms | .23 |

*Note.* n of patients in this investigaiton = 150. Patient ratings were made by each patient's primary therapist following the fourth psychotherapy session. All correlations in this table are significant at $p < .05$. Adapted from Lorr and McNair (1964b, Tables 1 and 2). © 1964 by Williams and Wilkins. Adapted by permission of the publisher.

Thus, Lorr and McNair's (1964b) findings parallel O'Neill and Bornstein's (1990) results regarding the relationship of dependency to help-seeking response set on the MMPI. In addition, these findings are consistent with the results of numerous studies (described in detail in Chapter 4) that demonstrated that dependency is associated with increased frequencies of help-seeking behaviors in a variety of social settings. Lorr and McNair's findings also support the clinical observations of Emery and Lesher (1982): Consistent with Emery and Lesher's observations (described earlier), Lorr and McNair found that dependency is associated with both positive and negative behaviors during psychotherapy.

## Dependency and Treatment Duration

Several studies indicate that dependent individuals remain in treatment longer than do nondependent individuals, presumably because the dependent person is reluctant to relinquish the patient–caretaker relationship. Of the three studies that examined the dependency–treatment relationship in hospitalized patients, two (Brown & Rawlinson, 1975; Greenberg & Bornstein, 1989) found a significant positive correlation between the patient's level of dependency and duration of the hospital stay, while one investigation (Overholser et al., 1989) found only a weak relationship between these variables. Although results in this area have been somewhat inconsistent, it appears that a significant positive relationship between dependency and length of inpatient hospital treatment is found in both men and women, and for both medical illnesses (i.e., cardiac surgery; Brown & Rawlinson, 1975) and psychiatric disorders (Greenberg & Bornstein, 1989).

The effect of patient dependency on length of hospital stay is not only statistically significant but also quite substantial. Greenberg and Bornstein (1989) found that dependent female psychiatric patients (assessed via the ROD scale) remained in a voluntary treatment unit nearly twice as long as did nondependent female patients: Mean length of stay was 101 days for dependent patients versus 60 days for nondependent patients. In light of (1) the tremendous financial costs associated with inpatient psychiatric treatment and (2) recent efforts to reduce the costs associated with treating various physical and psychiatric disorders, these findings have important practical as well as theoretical significance (see Chapter 10 for a detailed discussion of this issue).

Although the majority of studies of the dependency–treatment duration relationship in hospitalized patients produced positive results, studies of the dependency–treatment duration relationship in outpatients have yielded more mixed findings. Of the four studies that examined the dependency–treatment duration relationship in outpatients, two investigations (Snyder, 1963; Stamler & Palmer, 1971) obtained the predicted pattern of results, but two investigations (Hiler, 1959; Lorr & McNair, 1964a) obtained nonsignificant findings. On the positive side, Snyder found a correlation of .36 between level of dependency and duration of psychotherapy in a sample of 20 adult outpatients, while Stamler and Palmer obtained a correlation of .29 between level of dependency and the duration of outpatient treatment for physical illness in a mixed-sex sample of 34 elementary school children. On the negative side, Hiler obtained a nonsignificant correlation ($r = .03$) between level of dependency and the duration of outpatient psychotherapy in a sample of 70 adult patients, while Lorr and McNair obtained a nonsignificant correlation ($r = .09$) between level of dependency and duration of psychotherapy in a large multicenter study involving more than 200 therapists and 500 psychotherapy patients.

In retrospect, it is not surprising that the dependency–treatment duration relationship is somewhat stronger for inpatient than outpatient treatment. Without question, terminating inpatient treatment entails a greater shift toward independence on the part of the patient than does terminating outpatient treatment. In this respect, relinquishing the patient–therapist (or patient–physician) relationship is likely to be more difficult for the dependent person in an inpatient setting than for the dependent person in an outpatient setting. Of course, one could make the argument that termination of outpatient psychotherapy is in some ways more "permanent" than termination of inpatient treatment. After all, hospital discharge is typically followed by some period of outpatient psychotherapy, which allows the patient–therapist relationship to continue after inpatient treatment has ended. However, while the patient–therapist relationship often continues after the patient is discharged from the hospital, this relationship is considerably less intense (and involves much less day-to-day contact) when it is continued on an outpatient basis. In any case, it is clear that—for whatever reason—the dependency–treatment duration relationship holds primarily for inpatient psychiatric and medical treatment.

The results of one additional investigation warrant brief discussion in the present context. Salokangas, Rakkolainen, and Lehtinen (1980) conducted a large-scale longitudinal study of posthospitalization adjustment in a mixed-sex sample of 75 schizophrenic patients. At the outset of the study, the patients were divided into four groups with respect to their dependency-related attitudes and behaviors: (1) highly dependent; (2) nondependent; (3) situationally dependent (i.e., exhibiting situation-appropriate dependent and nondependent behaviors at different times); and (4) denying dependency (i.e., refusing to acknowledge any dependent feelings or motivations whatsoever). Salokangas et al. (1980) took repeated follow-up measures of adjustment from each patient for an 8-year period following the patient's initial inpatient treatment for schizophrenia.

Salokangas et al. (1980) found that—as predicted—the initial dependency ratings predicted patients' subsequent treatment-related behaviors. Specifically, the dependent patients remained in outpatient psychotherapy throughout most of the follow-up period but had relatively few rehospitalizations. In contrast, the nondependent and situationally dependent patients spent less time in outpatient treatment than did the dependent patients. Finally, the patients classified as denying dependency showed the lowest overall incidence of follow-up treatment. Although this study used very different procedures and measures than were used by Greenberg and Bornstein (1989) in their study of dependency and treatment duration (described earlier), Salokangas et al.'s (1980) results are nonetheless consistent with those of Bornstein and Greenberg (1989): In both investigations, high levels of dependency were associated with an inability (or unwillingness) to terminate treatment and leave the patient role.

## DEPENDENCY AND TREATMENT COMPLIANCE

Early studies of the dependency–treatment compliance relationship produced highly consistent results, finding that dependent medical patients are viewed by their physicians as being more compliant and cooperative than are nondependent patients (see Davis & Eichorn, 1963; Moran, Fairweather, Fisher, & Morton, 1956; Vernier, Barroll, Cummings, Dickerson, & Cooper, 1961). Unfortunately, these investigations are characterized by three important methodological limitations. First, studies in this area all relied on subjective reports of patient compliance rather than utilizing objective compliance measures. Thus, it is difficult to know to what degree the physicians' reports obtained in these investigations reflect a general positive attitude toward the dependent patient, and to what degree these reports reflect accurately different patients' levels of compliance with treatment regimens. As Greenberg and Fisher (1977) and others have noted, physicians typically prefer compliant, passive patients over independent, assertive patients.

A second methodological limitation of these studies involves the way in which dependency was assessed. Typically, the physicians who provided ratings of patient compliance in these investigations also provided ratings of patient dependency. Thus, it is possible that physicians' ratings of patient dependency and patient compliance were not completely independent, so that a "halo effect" occurred, and ratings of dependency were based—in whole or in part—on compliant behavior exhibited by patients in the medical setting (see Chapter 2 for a discussion of similar methodological problems in observer ratings of dependent classroom behavior in children).

A third limitation of studies of the dependency–compliance relationship in patients involves the limited range of patient subjects who have been assessed in these investigations thus far. Specifically, it is unfortunate that—as was the case in studies of the dependency–treatment delay relationship—studies of the dependency–compliance relationship have focused exclusively on dependency and compliance in medical patients. Consequently, the degree to which dependency predicts compliance and cooperativeness in hospitalized psychiatric patients remains unknown.

Although there have been no studies of the dependency–compliance relationship in psychiatric inpatients, two recent investigations (Nacev, 1980; Poldrugo & Forti, 1988) examined the relationship of patient dependency to objective measures of compliance with outpatient psychological treatment. These investigations produced conflicting results. In Nacev's study, 100 adult outpatients (50 men and 50 women) completed MMPI protocols, from which Dy scores were derived. Records of each patient's attendance in weekly psychotherapy sessions (i.e., the number of sessions missed but not canceled beforehand) were kept by their primary therapist. There was a small (but nonsignificant) correlation between dependency score and number of missed sessions ($r = -.13$), with dependent patients missing fewer psychotherapy sessions than nondependent patients.

Poldrugo and Forti (1988) obtained much stronger results in their study of dependency and compliance with outpatient treatment for alcoholism. In this investigation, structured diagnostic interviews were administered to 717 male patients initiating voluntary outpatient psychotherapy; of these, 102 (25%) received diagnoses of an Axis II personality disorder. Poldrugo and Forti then compared treatment compliance rates (defined as "consistent attendance" in group therapy sessions throughout the 1-year period following the initiation of treatment) among patients with different personality disorder diagnoses. As predicted, DPD patients showed significantly higher rates of treatment compliance than did patients in any other group. Overall, 75% of DPD patients (versus 33% of non-DPD patients) completed the 1-year course of treatment and remained abstinent for the duration of the study.

The conflicting results obtained by Nacev (1980) and Poldrugo and Forti (1988) may be due to differences in the way that treatment compliance was operationalized in these two investigations. In Nacev's study, treatment compliance was defined as the number of psychotherapy sessions missed, while in Poldrugo and Forti's study, compliance was defined as completion of a 1-year alcohol abuse treatment regimen. It is impossible to say which of these measures of treatment compliance is more valid. However, it is clear that they are assessing different categories of behavior. Nacev's operational definition of treatment compliance focused only on patient cooperativeness and compliance during the course of treatment, while Poldrugo and Forti's operational definition of treatment compliance focused exclusively on the successful completion of a treatment program.

Thus, comparison of the results obtained in these two investigations suggests that the relationship between dependency and treatment compliance—if it exists—is likely to be manifest primarily in terms of treatment follow-through (i.e., completion of treatment regimens), rather than in day-to-day compliance with treatment.

## DEPENDENCY, PERCEPTIONS OF THE PSYCHOTHERAPIST, AND PSYCHOTHERAPY PREFERENCE

Because research in this area has consisted almost entirely of isolated, unreplicated studies, the degree to which strong conclusions can be drawn from these findings is limited. Nonetheless, these results are generally consistent with other findings regarding the behavior of dependent persons in social and clinical settings and suggest that dependent individuals (1) have more positive attitudes regarding psychotherapy (and psychotherapists) than do nondependent individuals (Heller & Goldstein, 1961; Lorr & McNair, 1964b); (2) make more accurate inferences regarding the therapist's attitudes and personal beliefs than do nondependent persons (Masling et al., 1980); and (3) prefer psychodynamic treatment over forms of therapy that involve a less intense patient–therapist relationship (Juni & LoCascio, 1985).

In an early study in this area, Heller and Goldstein (1961) obtained a significant positive correlation ($r = .50$) between level of dependency (assessed by self-report and via a behavioral dependency measure) and the degree to which psychotherapy was perceived in a positive manner in a mixed-sex sample of 30 psychiatric outpatients. Lorr and McNair (1964b) subsequently obtained similar but weaker results in a sample of 150 male outpatients. These results are consistent with Zeldow and Greenberg's (1979, 1980) findings (discussed earlier) that dependent women report more positive attitudes regarding physicians and hospitals than do nondependent women. Presumably, being involved in an ongoing relationship with a powerful caretaker is gratifying to the dependent person.

Along different lines, Masling et al. (1980) followed up on Masling et al.'s (1974) study of dependency and accuracy of perceptions of roommates and acquaintances by investigating the relationship of dependency to accuracy of perceptions of the therapist. Using a methodology similar to that of their initial 1974 study (see Chapter 4 for a detailed description of this investigation), Masling et al. (1980) assessed level of dependency in 21 adult psychotherapy patients by calculating each patient's ROD score from Rorschach protocols that had been administered during the intake process. Following the third therapy session, and again immediately following termination of therapy, patients completed a questionnaire that required them to make a series of ratings of their therapist's political beliefs, personal interests, and attitudes regarding various social issues. Consistent with the earlier findings of Masling et al. (1974) for acquaintances and roommates, Masling et al. (1980) found that dependent patients gave more accurate responses than did nondependent patients when judging their therapist's attitudes and beliefs.

Finally, Juni and LoCascio (1985) examined dependent and nondependent persons' preferences for different types of psychotherapy. In this study, a mixed-sex sample of undergraduates was divided into dependent and nondependent groups based on their ROD scores. Subjects were then given a set of descriptions of different types of psychotherapy (i.e., psychoanalytic, client centered, cognitive–behavioral), and were asked to rate on a 10-point scale their likelihood of choosing each form of therapy if they ever sought psychological treatment. Juni and LoCascio hypothesized that dependent individuals would prefer psychoanalytic therapy over other forms of therapy because they would perceive psychoanalysis as affording a greater amount of contact with the therapist and a more "intimate" therapeutic relationship. This hypothesis was confirmed. Dependent subjects of both sexes preferred psychoanalytic therapy over other forms of therapy (although Juni & LoCascio did not obtain information regarding the reasoning behind the subjects' decisions). Despite the fact that this study employed undergraduates rather than clinical subjects, Juni and LoCascio's results nonetheless suggest that preference for psychotherapy may be influenced by a person's level of dependency.[1]

## NOTE

1. Interestingly, Juni and LoCascio's (1985) findings are in some ways consistent with Benfari's (1969) cross-cultural study of dependency and patient–healer relationships. Benfari found a strong positive relationship between the degree to which a particular culture indulged childhood dependency behavior and the degree to which healers (e.g., physicians, shamans) in that culture (1) adopted a "person-oriented" approach to treatment and (2) were viewed as omniscient, onmipotent figures (see also Parker [1960] for additional anthropological evidence bearing on this issue).

# The Dependent Personality: Toward an Integrated Theoretical Model

In light of the wide variety of topics examined by dependency researchers, and the different subject groups, experimental procedures, and dependency measures used in different studies, the degree to which developmental, social, and clinical investigations of dependency have produced consistent results is remarkable. Parallel findings have emerged in a number of important areas (e.g., with respect to the behavior of dependent individuals in social and clinical settings, with respect to the role of interpersonal stress as a risk factor for depression and physical illness in dependent persons). Moreover, studies involving subjects from different cultures (i.e., American, British, Canadian, Indian, Italian, German, Japanese, Israeli, Hungarian, Austrian, Australian, Norwegian, Belgian, Dutch) have produced highly consistent findings (e.g., research on parenting style, sex role, suggestibility, interpersonal compliance, help seeking, affiliative behavior, performance anxiety, jealousy, sociometric status, depression, phobias, alcoholism, and physical disorders).

Not only is there a great deal of cross-cultural consistency in the findings that have emerged in empirical studies of the dependent personality, there is also considerable cross-gender consistency in these findings. Similar results were obtained for men and women in most areas of dependency research (e.g., in studies of parenting style, suggestibility, interpersonal compliance, help seeking, verbal conditioning, affiliative behavior, performance anxiety, jealousy, phobias, smoking, ulcers, cancer, and behavior in clinical settings). In two areas (i.e., interpersonal sensitivity and depression), findings were somewhat stronger for men than for women.

I hesitate to make too much of the slightly stronger effects obtained for men in these two areas of dependency research because in both of these areas men and women produced similar patterns of results. However, the stronger effects obtained for men in studies of the dependency–depression and dependency–interpersonal sensitivity relationships may well be due to the effects of cultural attitudes and beliefs regarding dependency on the overt expression of dependent behavior in men and women. As discussed in Chapters 1 and 3, dependency is viewed as a "feminine" trait in most Western societies (see Ashmore, 1981; Cadbury, 1991; Mischel, 1970; Spence & Helmreich, 1978). Consequently, while men are discouraged from expressing or acknowledging dependent feelings, women have historically been encouraged to express such feelings openly. Thus, overt dependent behavior is less common in men than in women, and dependency in men is a more "unusual" and noteworthy trait than is dependency in women. In this context, it is not surprising that dependency in men is a slightly better predictor of certain traits and behaviors than is dependency in women.

Finally, there is substantial cross-measure and cross-methodology consistency in the results obtained in studies of the dependent personality. In fact, in *every* area of research where studies have used both oral dependency scales and measures of interpersonal dependency, the two types of measures have yielded highly similar findings. Moreover, with the exception of the well-established finding that objective dependency measures yield greater sex differences than do projective dependency measures, these two types of measures have invariably produced consistent results in developmental, social, and clinical studies of the dependent personality.

Overall, the picture of the dependent person that emerges from this review is considerably more complex than one might expect based on the traditional psychological view of dependency. The vast majority of theoreticians and researchers have focused primarily on the negative consequences of dependent personality traits (see Ainsworth, 1969; Birtchnell, 1988a; Millon, 1981). Consistent with this viewpoint, the research reviewed in this book confirms that dependency is associated with a number of "negative" traits (e.g., suggestibility, conformity, jealousy), with increased risk for physical illness, and with risk for certain psychological disorders (e.g., depression, tobacco addiction). However, dependency is also associated with such positive traits as the ability to infer accurately the attitudes and beliefs of other people (i.e., interpersonal sensitivity), a desire to perform well in psychology experiments, and a tendency to seek medical attention quickly when physical symptoms appear. Thus, instead of being simply a problem, deficit, or flaw, as many researchers have suggested, dependency is associated with both positive and negative qualities.

# TOWARD AN INTEGRATED THEORETICAL MODEL OF DEPENDENCY

In Chapter 1, I offered a tentative working definition of dependency that included four components: cognitive, affective, motivational, and behavioral. Because this was intended to be a working definition of dependency rather than a definitive model, I did not specify the relationships among these four hypothesized components, nor was I very specific regarding the particular features of each component of the working definition. Now that I have discussed in detail the results of several hundred empirical studies in this area, I am in a position to be more specific regarding the components of the dependent personality.

The studies reviewed in Chapters 3 through 9 offer strong support for the four basic features of the working definition of dependency described in Chapter 1. Clearly, cognitive, affective, and motivational factors all play a role in determining the behavior of dependent persons in various situations and settings. The studies reviewed in this book also allow me to draw some tentative conclusions regarding the relationships among these (and other) components of the dependent personality. In some cases, causal relationships among particular variables have been clearly established by the converging results of well-designed empirical studies. In other cases, there is evidence that suggests particular patterns of relationships, but this evidence is not definitive. In formulating an integrated model of dependency, I have included both well-established findings and more tentative, speculative relationships. I will try to point out which components of the model are strongly supported by the results of relevant empirical studies and which components of the model are more tentative. Ultimately, though, the validity of the model must be established (or refuted) by future experiments.

The basic features of an integrated theoretical model of dependency are presented in Figure 10.1. The arrows in Figure 10.1 represent causal relationships among different variables, with the direction of causality indicated by the direction of the arrows. In the following sections, I expand and elaborate on the most important components of the model.

## The Etiology of Dependency

As Figure 10.1 shows, the etiology of individual differences in childhood and adult dependency lies in two areas: overprotective, authoritarian parenting and sex-role socialization. The effects of these two processes on the etiology and dynamics of dependency were discussed in detail in Chapter 3. Broadly speaking, individual differences in parenting style may be regarded as a "family-specific" influence on dependency, while sex-role socialization

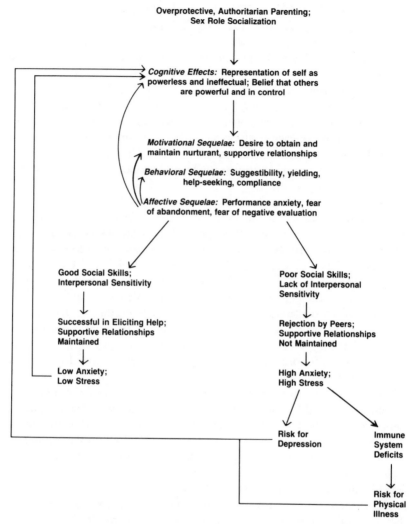

**FIGURE 10.1.** An integrated theoretical model of dependency.

experiences represent a more general, culture-bound influence on the acquisition and development of dependent personality traits. Having said this, I can be more specific regarding the nature of these two hypothesized etiological factors, and regarding the ways in which these two factors interact to determine level of dependency in children and adults. I will briefly discuss four issues regarding the effects of parenting practices and sex-role socialization experiences on dependency.

First, it is important to note that parenting style and sex-role socialization practices are not completely independent. A great deal of sex-role socialization (especially early socialization) takes place within the family. Moreover, it is likely that global indices of parenting style predict important aspects of a parent's sex-role socialization practices. For example, research indicates that highly authoritarian parents tend to encourage traditional sex-role-related behaviors in their children to a greater degree than do less authoritarian parents (see Baumrind, 1971; Maccoby, 1980). This turns out to have very different implications for boys and girls. In young girls, authoritarian parenting practices and traditional sex-role socialization experiences will tend to work in concert to promote dependent behavior. In young boys, the interactive effects of authoritarian parenting practices and traditional sex-role socialization experiences are more complicated in that authoritarian parents will be likely to encourage sex-role-typed behaviors in boys, while simultaneously engaging in the kinds of authoritarian parenting practices that discourage independent decision making and autonomous behavior.

Second, although I did not include any reference to infantile feeding and weaning practices in this first component of the model, it is certainly possible that these practices influence a child's level of dependency. As noted in Chapter 3, it is likely that certain feeding and weaning practices that potentially play a role in determining level of dependency (e.g., rigidity of feeding schedule) are systematically related to parenting style, but this relationship has not yet been demonstrated conclusively.

Third, although research has demonstrated that overprotective, authoritarian parenting practices play a role in the etiology of dependency, it is not clear whether there is a "critical period" during which these parenting practices must be exhibited in order to produce high levels of dependency in the child. The methodologies used in studies of the dependency–parenting style relationship that have been conducted to date do not allow firm conclusions to be drawn regarding this issue. It is reasonable to postulate that high levels of dependency are particularly likely to result when overprotective, authoritarian parenting practices (1) begin early; (2) are exhibited consistently across different situations; and (3) remain relatively constant as the child ages. However, the degree to which the early onset, cross-situational consistency and temporal stability of overprotective, authoritarian parenting practices actually influence the acquisition and development of dependent personality traits in children is an empirical question that has not yet been addressed.

Finally, by placing "parenting" at the top of my model, I have avoided an important question: Why do some parents treat their children in an overprotective and/or authoritarian manner while other parents treat their children very differently? One possibility is that parental overprotectiveness and authoritarianism resides entirely within the parents. In other words, it is possible that the personalities of the parents are the sole determinant of their parenting style. While this is certainly possible—and is undoubtedly true in at least some cases—this explanation seems overly simplistic, and inadequate as an explanation of most parents' childrearing practices. The fact is that parents and children form dyads (and triads) whose individual members interact and influence each others' behavior (see Beebe [1986] for a summary of research in this area). Moreover, as discussed in Chapter 3, it is clear that some temperament-related behaviors exhibited by the infant (e.g., adaptability, soothability) play a role in determining the parents' approach to childrearing. These temperament variables may also have a direct influence on the development of dependent behaviors in children (see Chapter 3 for a detailed discussion of this issue).[1]

Sears et al. (1957) captured nicely the "chicken and egg" paradox that confronts theoreticians and researchers who wrestle with this question. Sears et al. (1957) noted:

> [We are] skeptical that there is any single direction of cause-and-effect relations in the child-rearing process. True, the mother's personality comes first chronologically, and she starts the sequence of interactive behavior that culminates in the child's personality. But once a child starts to be overdependent—or is *perceived* as being so by his mother—he becomes a stimulus to the mother and influences her behavior toward him. . . . The whole relationship [becomes] circular. An enormous amount of painstaking research will be required to untangle these phenomena. (p. 175)

Thirty-five years after Sears et al.'s (1957) call for research examining more closely the relationship of individual differences in children's dependency to individual differences in caretaker behavior, developmental researchers have still not disentangled completely the relationship between these variables.

## The Cognitive, Motivational, Behavioral, and Affective Sequelae of Overprotective, Authoritarian Parenting

Without question, overprotective, authoritarian parenting will have several effects on the child's dependency-related thoughts, feelings, and behaviors. In my view, the most immediate consequences of overprotective, authoritarian parenting will be (1) the construction of particular mental representations of the self and other people and (2) the acquisition of particular beliefs regarding one's own self-efficacy and regarding the power and potency of others.[2] Specifically, because early relationships with the parents play a central role in the construction of the self-concept, the children of overprotective parents will come to believe that they cannot function adequately without the guidance and protection of others, particularly figures of authority (Millon, 1981; Parker, 1983). Furthermore, because early relationships with the parents create particular expectations for future interpersonal relationships (Blatt, 1974; Waters & Deane, 1985), parental overprotectiveness will lead to an expectation on the part of children that they will be nurtured and cared for by others. Similarly, parental authoritarianism will lead children to believe that the way to maintain good relationships with others is to acquiesce to their requests, expectations, and demands (Baumrind, 1973; Kaul et al., 1982).

Thus, cognitive structures (i.e., self and object representations) that are formed in response to early experiences within the family will influence the motivations, behaviors, and affective responses of the dependent person in predictable ways. A perception of oneself as powerless and in need of guidance and support from others will, first and foremost, have motivational effects. A person with such a self-concept will be motivated to seek guidance, support, protection, and nurturance from other people. These self-concept-based motivations in turn produce particular patterns of dependent behavior: The person who is highly motivated to seek the guidance, protection, and support of others will behave in ways that maximize the probability that they will obtain the guidance, protection, and support that they desire. Finally, a representation of the self as powerless and ineffectual will have important affective consequences (e.g., fear of abandonment, performance anxiety, fear of negative evaluation).

Although cognitive structures produced in response to early parenting and socialization experiences mediate the motivations, behaviors, and affective responses of the dependent person, I believe that affective responses come to play a particularly important role in the dynamics of dependency. As Figure 10.1 shows, affective responses systematically influence the cognitions, motivations, and behaviors of the dependent person. Specifically, dependency-related affective responses (e.g., performance anxiety) strengthen and reinforce dependency-related motivations (e.g., need for support). That is, when a stimulus or situation stimulates a dependency-related affective response, the individual's dependency-related motivations will increase. Similarly, when a dependency-related affective response is stimulated, dependent behavior is more likely to be exhibited. Most important, though, dependency-related affective responses strengthen and reinforce the dependent person's belief in their own ineffectiveness and powerlessness. Thus, a feedback loop is formed wherein affective responses that initially resulted from particular beliefs regarding the self and others ultimately come to reinforce and strengthen those very same beliefs (see Figure 10.1). Similar feedback loops characterize the affect–motivation and affect–behavior relationships.

## The "Core" Motivation of the Dependent Person

Ironically, although one might suppose that the dependent person's internalized self and object representations would invariably lead him or her to behave in a passive, compliant manner toward others, this turns out not to be the case. To be sure, the behavior of the dependent person is often characterized by passivity and compliance. However, the prevailing view of dependent individuals as uniformly passive and compliant is clearly contradicted by the findings discussed in this book. In certain situations (e.g., when placed in the role of "medical patient" or when asked to serve as a subject in a psychology experiment), dependency is indeed associated with passivity and compliance. However, in other situations, the dependent person is anything but passive. Studies confirm that dependent individuals ask for feedback on psychological tests more readily than do nondependent persons (Juni, 1981), ask for help when attempting to solve difficult problems in the laboratory more frequently than do nondependent persons (Shilkret & Masling, 1981), and seek medical attention more quickly than do nondependent persons when physical symptoms appear (Greenberg & Fisher, 1977). Although these behaviors are all characterized by help seeking, they are also characterized by an assertive, active stance.

How can we reconcile the seemingly inconsistent findings that dependent individuals are passive and acquiescent in certain contexts and active and assertive in others? We can do this by examining in more detail the motivations that underlie the dependent individual's behavior in different situations. The results of studies reviewed in Chapters 3 through 9 suggest that one central goal underlies much of the dependent person's behavior: obtaining and maintaining nurturant, supportive relationships. This "core" motivation of the dependent person is reflected in a wide variety of situations and settings, albeit in different ways. Thus, the dependent person yields to group pressure in most situations (Masling et al., 1968), except when doing so might displease a figure of authority (Bornstein et al., 1987). The dependent person is cooperative in experimental (Bornstein & Masling, 1985), medical (Davis & Eichorn, 1963), and psychiatric settings (Poldrugo & Forti, 1988), shows high levels of performance anxiety (Ojha, 1978), and is responsive to subtle interpersonal cues emitted by peers (Masling et al., 1974), experimenters (Weiss, 1969), teachers (Juni & Semel, 1982), and therapists (Masling et al., 1980). Termination—or the perceived threat of termination—of important interpersonal relationships not only increases the dependent person's level of depression (Hammen et al., 1985) but appears to place her at risk for a variety of physical illnesses as well (Greenberg & Bornstein, 1988a).

Given dependent persons' strong motivation to obtain and maintain supportive relationships, the apparent inconsistency in their behavior across different situations is easy to understand. Dependent individuals simply choose to exhibit behaviors that they believe will maximize their chances of obtaining and maintaining such relationships. When passive, compliant behavior seems likely to achieve this goal, the dependent person chooses to act in a passive manner. When assertive, active behavior seems more likely to achieve this goal, the dependent person becomes active and assertive. Exhibiting passive, compliant behavior in certain situations and active help-seeking behavior in others merely represents an attempt on the part of the dependent person to fulfill the underlying goal of obtaining and maintaining the supportive, protective relationships that they so strongly desire.[3]

Thus, the compliant behavior that is sometimes exhibited by the dependent person is best understood not as genuine passivity and lack of assertiveness, but rather as a kind of self-presentation strategy that is intended to make certain kinds of impressions on others in order to achieve specific goals. As Jones and Pittman (1982) noted, "by stressing his inability to fend for himself and emphasizing his dependence on others, the [dependent individual] makes salient a norm of obligation or social responsibility" (p. 247). The research reviewed in Chapter 5 confirms that passive, dependent behaviors do in fact serve as social cues that elicit supportive and helping responses from other people (see, e.g., Baker & Reitz, 1978; Barnes et al., 1979; Berkowitz & Daniels, 1963, 1964). Apparently, the dependent person knows that exhibiting passive, helpless behavior can, in certain situations, be a useful way of obtaining help and support. Whether this knowledge is implicit (and hence, unverbalizable) or explicit (and hence, accessible to conscious awareness) is an empirical question that has not been addressed.

The hypothesis that the dependent person's "core" motivation is to obtain and maintain nurturant, protective relationships is consistent with the finding that overprotective, authoritarian parenting predicts level of dependency in childhood, adolescence, and adulthood. I will have more to say about that issue in the following section. For the time being, we can turn to the model depicted in Figure 10.1 to illustrate the connection between early parenting experiences and the "core" motivation of the dependent person. Working backwards through the model, it is clear that the behaviors exhibited by the dependent person in social and clinical settings reflect the "core" motivation of the dependent individual, which may be traced to particular beliefs about the self and other people, which in turn may be traced to early experiences within the family.[4]

## Long-Term Consequences of Dependency

Masling et al.'s (1974, 1980) findings regarding the relationship of dependency to interpersonal sensitivity suggest that, as a group, dependent persons tend to be highly skilled at decoding subtle interpersonal cues. Regardless of whether these results generalize to the entire population of dependent individuals, two implications of Masling et al.'s findings are noteworthy in the present context. First, research suggests that interpersonal sensitivity and level of social skill covary, with individuals who are sensitive to interpersonal cues generally showing better social skills than individuals who are less sensitive to interpersonal cues (see Aronson, 1992; Caspi et al., 1989). Second, despite the fact that there may be a positive relationship between level of dependency and degree of social skill, it is clear that some dependent persons have better social skills than others. In other words, it should be possible to divide any group of dependent individuals into those with "good social skills" and those with "poor social skills," even if dependent individuals as a group tend to cluster at the "good social skills" end of the continuum.

Because the "core" motivation of the dependent person is to obtain and maintain nurturant, supportive relationships, the degree to which a dependent individual has acquired good social skills (including sensitivity to interpersonal cues) will have important implications for the long-term consequences of dependency. In Figure 10.1, I have arbitrarily divided the population of dependent persons into those with "good social skills" and those with "poor social skills" in order to illustrate the effects of this variable on the long-term consequences of dependency. I will briefly discuss the hypothesized effects of good versus poor social skills on the long-term consequences of dependency, beginning with the population of dependent persons who *are* socially skilled. This group is designated by the lefthand arrow in the middle of Figure 10.1.

As Figure 10.1 shows, good social skills should be associated with success in eliciting social support (Berkowitz, 1972; Daniels & Berkowitz, 1963) and with the ability to obtain and maintain supportive, nurturant relationships (see Caspi et al., 1989). In fact, the effects of good social skills and high levels of interpersonal sensitivity on an individual's ability to obtain and maintain good interpersonal relationships will be threefold. First, interpersonal sensitivity should help the dependent person to *identify* those individuals who are likely to meet their needs for nurturance, guidance, and support. Second, good social skills should enable the dependent person to *develop* relationships with potential nurturers and protectors. Third, good social skills and sensitivity to interpersonal cues should enable the dependent person to *maintain* good relationships with these nurturers and protectors.

To the extent that dependent persons are able to obtain and maintain the supportive relationships that they desire, anxiety and stress should be minimized. In a sense, this represents the best possible long-term outcome of dependency. However, two less-than-positive consequences of this long-term outcome are worth mentioning. First, the dependent person in this situation has, in effect, recapitulated the earlier parent–child relationship that led to his dependency in the first place. In other words, the dependent person has sought out a guide/protector who functions much like the overprotective, authoritarian parent of infancy and childhood. Second, insofar as the presence of a nurturant, supportive other serves as an anxiety and stress reducer for the dependent person, the presence of a nurturer/protector will serve to reinforce the dependent person's "helpless" self-concept. In other words, to the extent that the dependent person continues to rely on a significant other for guidance, protection, and support, the dependent individual will continue to believe that he or she cannot function independently, without the protection and help of others.

The dependent individual with less effective social skills will not be as successful in obtaining and maintaining supportive, protective relationships. This will lead to a very different—and less positive—long-term outcome. This outcome is depicted on the righthand side of Figure 10.1. As this part of Figure 10.1 shows, poor social skills will lead to an absence of supportive, nurturant relationships, which in turn will lead to increased anxiety and stress for the dependent person. This increased anxiety and stress has implications for both psychological and physical adjustment. With respect to psychological functioning, high levels of stress and anxiety will lead to increased risk for depression (and possibly eating disorders) in the dependent individual (see Chapter 6 for a detailed discussion of the dependency–stress–psychopathology relationship). With respect to physiological functioning, high levels of anxiety and stress may lead to diminished immunocompetence in the dependent person, ultimately leading to increased risk for various physical illnesses that are mediated by immune system functioning (see Chapter 8 for a discussion of empirical evidence bearing on this issue).

Finally, the onset of physical or psychological illness will have implications for the dependent person's behavior and self-concept. As discussed in Chapters 8 and 9, the onset of illness is typically followed by an increase in dependent, help-seeking behavior. In addition, to the extent that the dependent person assumes the "sick role" following the onset of physical or psychological illness, her perception of herself as powerless, ineffectual, and dependent on others for support and protection will increase.

Thus, it is ironic that while interpersonal sensitivity and good social skills appear to play a critical role in determining the long-term outcome of dependency, both of the possible long-term outcomes depicted in Figure 10.1 lead to the same end: reinforcement of the dependent person's "helpless" self-concept. In a sense, this conclusion is not surprising. Numerous studies have demonstrated that individuals typically behave (and process social and self-referent information) in such a way as to "protect" and reinforce preexisting beliefs about the self and other people (see Kihlstrom

& Cantor, 1984; Snyder, 1981). In this context, Caspi et al. (1989) suggested:

> [D]ependency as an individual interactional style may well be even more
> self-perpetuating than [other personality styles] because dependent individuals
> are positively motivated to select and construct environments that sustain their
> dependency. . . . [D]ependent persons recruit and attach themselves to others
> who will continue to provide the nurturance and support they seek. [Further-
> more], these individuals become increasingly skilled at evoking from others
> those nurturing responses that reinforce their dependency. (p. 395)

The conclusion that dependent individuals behave in such a way as to
propogate their "helpless" self-concept and maintain preexisting relationship and behavior patterns is certainly consistent with the findings discussed
in previous chapters of this book. Moreover, this conclusion is also consistent with findings from empirical studies that describe efforts to increase
independent behavior in dependent persons via modeling, role playing, or
more typical therapeutic interventions such as pharmacological, behavioral,
or insight-oriented treatment (see Crowder, 1972; Jones, Wells, & Torrey,
1958; Lauer, 1976; Pandey, 1977; Rottschafer & Renzaglia, 1962; Saha &
Sinha, 1973; Snyder, 1963; Turkat & Carlson, 1984; Winder, Ahmad,
Bandura, & Rau, 1962). In most of these investigations, clinicians and
researchers have found that such interventions had little success in changing
the dependent individual's self-concept or long-term behavior.

## THE FUTURE OF DEPENDENCY RESEARCH

The integrated theoretical model of dependency depicted in Figure 10.1
suggests numerous avenues for future research on the dependent personality. I will not attempt to provide an exhaustive list of those research
possibilities here, but will leave it to the interested reader to draw his or her
own conclusions regarding the heuristic value of the model. In the following sections, I discuss a few directions for future research on dependency
and the dependent personality, some of which are closely tied to the model
depicted in Figure 10.1, and some of which stem from empirical findings
that were discussed in earlier chapters.

### Beyond the Traditional Dispositional
### Approach to Dependency

Because qualities of internalized self and object representations provide a
parsimonious explanation for the disparate behaviors exhibited by dependent persons in different situations and settings, object relations theory may

prove to be an important framework for conceptualizing the etiology, dynamics, and correlates of dependency. Of course, a considerable amount of research on self and object representations has come from outside object relations theory (see Blatt & Homann, 1992; Kihlstrom & Cantor, 1984; Stern, 1987; Westen, 1991). However, object relations theory provides a potentially rich source of data regarding dependency and the dependent personality, and this potentially rich data source has remained largely untapped. Although there have been a few studies of dependent individuals' self-representations (e.g., Bornstein et al., 1988a) and of dependent persons' mental representations of the parents (e.g., Blatt, Wein, Chevron, & Quinlan, 1979), much remains to be done in this area. To the extent that the dependent person's mental representations of significant individuals (e.g., self, parents, peers, teachers, doctors, therapists) are elucidated, our ability to understand and predict the behavior of dependent individuals in different contexts is likely to increase.

Thus, it may be time to shift our attention to investigating the object-relational aspects of dependency. For better or worse, dependency research during the past 40 years has been dominated by classical psychoanalytic theory and by the social learning model. However, the results of studies reviewed in this book suggest that object-relational constructs represent important links among the disparate behaviors exhibited by dependent individuals in different situations and settings. Moreover, the object relations framework may provide important links between the psychoanalytic and social learning models of dependency. Object relations theory allows us to integrate some crucial psychoanalytic concepts (e.g., the importance of unconscious, unexpressed dependency needs) with concepts from the social learning model (e.g., the importance of socialization experiences in shaping children's attitudes toward—and feelings regarding—dependency).

The fact that beliefs and expectations regarding the self and others play a central role in directing the behavior of the dependent person suggests not only that object relations theory will be a useful framework for future research in this area, but also that the traditional dispositional view of dependency may be overly narrow and somewhat limited in its ability to predict the behavior of the dependent person in different situations. Although adult dependency is a stable personality "trait" (or more accurately, a stable set of interrelated traits), the behavior of the dependent person can only be understood completely with reference to the context in which it is exhibited. As discussed in an earlier section of this chapter, although the core underlying motivation of the dependent person remains constant, the behavior that is exhibited by the dependent person changes somewhat from situation to situation, reflecting (1) the individual's perceptions of the demands, expectations, and behavioral constraints that characterize a given situation; and (2) the individual's beliefs regarding which behaviors are most likely to produce the desired outcome given those demands, expectations, and situational constraints.

The results of studies reviewed in this book suggest that in order to understand more fully the behavior of the dependent person, we must utilize an interactionist approach rather than relying solely on the traditional trait-oriented models. Consistent with Mischel's (1973, 1979, 1984) view that the behavior of individuals is best understood as proactive and directed by beliefs and expectations regarding self and others, studies conducted to date suggest that the behavior of the dependent person can only be understood fully (and predicted accurately) with reference the the dependent individual's underlying cognitive constructs. As Dweck and Leggett (1988) noted, the explanatory power of dispositional variables "lies in their ability to predict what behaviors will be exhibited in various situations, not in their prediction that the same behavior will be exhibited across situations" (p. 270). Similarly, Mischel (1984) argued:

> [A] theory of personality structure does not require a person to be characterizable by high levels of pervasive cross-situational consistency in everything he or she does. . . . Instead of seeking high levels of consistency from situation to situation for many behaviors in a wide range of contexts, [we should] try to identify unique "bundles" or sets of temporally stable prototypic behaviors, key features, that characterize the person even over long periods of time but not necessarily across most or all possibly relevant situations. (p. 362)

Because dependent persons interpret different situations as involving different demands, opportunities, and risks, they choose to behave in somewhat different ways in different contexts. Underlying these surface differences in behavior, however, is a fundamental consistency: When the prototypic behaviors of the dependent individual in different situations and settings are interpreted in the context of the dependent person's most important cognitive constructs (i.e., a view of the self as powerless and ineffectual, and a belief that others can provide needed guidance and protection) and motivations (i.e., a desire to be guided and supported by others), apparent inconsistencies in the behaviors exhibited in different settings simply disappear.

## The Critical Importance of Dependency-Related Cognitions

In the integrated theoretical model of dependency depicted in Figure 10.1, dependency-related cognitions are the key determinant of the dependent person's motivations, behaviors, and affective responses. However, as noted in Chapter 1, the vast majority of studies of the dependent personality have come from developmental, social, and clinical psychology. When cognitive constructs are assessed in these studies, they are generally used only as a tool to investigate some developmental, social or clinical hypothesis (see, e.g., Blatt et al., 1979; Bornstein et al., 1986). In a sense, it is not surprising that there has been relatively little research on the cognitive correlates of dependency. With a few noteworthy exceptions (e.g., Abramson et al., 1978; Cacioppo & Petty, 1982), researchers have historically paid little attention to individual differences in cognitive "style." Thus, the absence of a cognitive psychology of dependency simply reflects the fact that researchers have not devoted a great deal of attention to developing a cognitive psychology of individual differences. Nonetheless, given the critical importance of dependency-related cognitions in determining the behavior of the dependent person in different situations and settings, it is time to develop a cognitive psychology of dependency.

In my view, a cognitive psychology of dependency must begin by examining in detail two issues that research suggests will be central to our understanding of the etiology and dynamics of dependent personality traits. First, as noted earlier, researchers must examine more fully the mental representations (i.e., cognitive schemata) of dependent individuals. These mental representations will not only provide important information regarding the etiology of dependency and help to integrate findings from the psychoanalytic and social learning models, but may also help to link ostensibly unrelated findings from developmental, social, and clinical studies of dependency.

Further investigation of the attributional correlates of dependency is also needed. To date, only two studies have examined directly the links between dependency and attributional style (Brewin & Furnham, 1987; Brown & Silberschatz, 1989). Although slightly different patterns of results were obtained in these two investigations, in both studies dependency was found to be associated with a "depressive" attributional style (i.e., a tendency to attribute the outcome of negative events to some internal cause while attributing the outcome of positive events to causes outside of one's control). Clearly, these results must be regarded as preliminary, and further research is needed to confirm and extend these initial findings. However, given the potential importance of the attributional correlates of dependency as mediators of goal-directed behaviors in different situations and settings, continued attention to this neglected topic is clearly warranted.

## Dependency as Diathesis

In light of the fact that one component of the dependent person's cognitive makeup is a dysfunctional attributional style, it is not surprising that the dependent person's cognitive constructs not only help to predict the dependent person's behavior in social and clinical settings, but also act as risk factors that—when coupled with events in the environment that exacerbate the individual's feelings of dependency and helplessness—place the dependent person at risk for physical and psychological disorders. In this respect, a dependent personality orientation may be conceptualized as a diathesis that combines with interpersonal stressors to predict the development of psychological and physical pathology.

The diathesis nature of dependency is most obvious in research on dependency and depression, and in studies of the relationship of dependency to risk for physical illness. In these two areas, it is clear that dependency and interpersonal stress (e.g., the disruption of important interpersonal relationships) combine to place the dependent person at risk for depression and disease. The extent to which this diathesis–stress framework predicts risk for other forms of psychopathology remains unknown. For example, although there is some indication that a similar diathesis–stress process may predict risk for eating disorders in dependent women, further research is needed to test this hypothesized relationship directly.

In any case, the dependent individual's cognitive makeup provides important clues regarding the relationship of dependency and interpersonal stress to risk for certain disorders. Clearly, a view of the self as powerless and ineffectual, coupled with a belief that others are comparatively powerful and in control of the outcome of situations, will lead the dependent person to attribute great importance to the disruption of important interpersonal relationships. Object relations theorists have long maintained that when important interpersonal relationships end or are threatened, the dependent person reexperiences early feelings of helplessness and infantile fears of abandonment by the primary caretaker (Blatt & Homann, 1992; Greenberg & Mitchell, 1983; Kernberg, 1976). Similar hypotheses have been put forth by social learning theorists, albeit in slightly different language (see Bandura, 1977; Dollard & Miller, 1950; Walters & Parke, 1964). Regardless of which theoretical framework one favors, it is clear that the dependent person's beliefs regarding self and others will cause him to experience the disruption or termination of important interpersonal relationships as extremely threatening and anxiety producing.

Although the most important diathesis aspect of dependency has to do with the dependent person's heightened vulnerability to interpersonal stress, dependency may act as a risk factor for psychopathology in another important way. Numerous studies have demonstrated that peer pressure and peer group affiliation play a central role in predicting risk for a variety of substance use disorders, including—but not limited to—tobacco and alcohol addiction (see Jessor & Jessor, 1977; Mosbach & Leventhal, 1988). Because dependent individuals are highly susceptible to interpersonal influence and tend to yield to group pressure in a variety of situations and settings, dependency may act as a diathesis for substance use disorders by increasing the dependent person's susceptibility to negative social influences from peers. In other words, if peer pressure plays a role in predicting adolescents' drug use behavior in general, it is likely that peer pressure will be a particularly strong risk factor for the dependent adolescent.

Of course, the dependent adolescent's susceptibility to social influence could also serve as protection from temptation to use tobacco, alcohol, or other drugs if at least one of two conditions are met. First, the dependent person's susceptibility to social influence will decrease the likelihood that he or she will use recreational drugs if the dependent person's peer group happens to frown on these activities. Second, dependency will decrease the likelihood of adolescent drug use if important authority figures in the dependent adolescent's life actively discourage drug use. In this situation, the dependent person is likely to be more strongly influenced by messages from authority figures than by peer pressure to use drugs (see Chapter 4, and the discussion of dependency and smoking in Chapter 6). Thus, dependency may represent a diathesis that increases risk for substance use disorders in certain situations, and as a strength that decreases risk for these disorders in other situations. Just as understanding the interpersonal context turned out to be important for predicting the behavior of the dependent person in social settings, it is clear that an understanding of the situation or context in which dependency is exhibited is critical for understanding the dependency–drug use relationship.

## From Theory to Application: Some Practical Implications of Dependency Research

Lewin (1951) once remarked that "there is nothing so practical as a good theory" (p. 169). That may be so, but it is also true that at some point a useful theory should generate empirical findings that have practical as well as theoretical value. Throughout this book, I have focused more or less exclusively on dependency theory and research, making little mention of potential applications of the findings obtained in this area. It is worthwhile to comment briefly on a few practical implications of dependency research.

The most obvious applications of dependency research involve medical and psychological treatment. Three sets of findings regarding the relationship of dependency to patient-related behaviors are particularly pertinent in this context. First, it is clear that dependency is associated with willingness to seek medical attention when somatic symptoms appear (Greenberg & Fisher, 1977). Second, several studies suggest that dependency predicts response to psychological treatment and may also predict recidivism following treatment (e.g., Fisher & Fisher, 1975; Mavissakalian & Hamann, 1987; Spolter et al., 1978). Third, the studies reviewed in Chapter 9 indicate that dependency is associated with an inability or unwillingness to relinquish the patient role following psychological and medical treatment (see, e.g., Brown & Rawlinson, 1975; Greenberg & Bornstein, 1989). In light of the ever-increasing costs of medical and psychological treatment, results in all three of these areas have important financial implications.

For example, consider Greenberg and Bornstein's (1989) finding that dependent female psychiatric inpatients remained hospitalized for an average of 40 days longer than members of a matched sample of nondependent female inpatients. Clearly, hospital costs vary considerably across different settings and locales, but suppose we estimate that inpatient psychiatric treatment at a particular setting averaged $350 per day (a ridiculously conservative estimate in this day and age). If that were the case, Greenberg and Bornstein's findings indicate that a dependent psychiatric inpatient would incur treatment costs that are at least $14,000 higher than those incurred by a nondependent psychiatric inpatient with a similar disorder.

Assessing level of dependency in medical and psychiatric patients on admission to the hospital would allow the treatment team to identify those patients who are likely to linger in the patient role. A dependent patient's treatment plan could then be structured in such a way that the patient was reinforced by figures of authority (e.g., the physician or therapist) for relinquishing aspects of the sick role in a timely manner. Moreover, in psychiatric settings, awareness of a patient's level of dependency—and the influence of exaggerated dependency needs on the termination and discharge process—would help the therapist to anticipate certain transference (and countertransference) reactions that might adversely affect treatment outcome (e.g., Davanloo, 1990; Emery & Lesher, 1982).

In a related vein, additional studies of the relationship between dependency and compliant, help-seeking behavior in clinical settings are likely to yield practical as well as theoretical gains. Given the dependent person's desire to please figures of authority, dependent individuals should comply with medical regimens more fully than will nondependent individuals. This should result in greater treatment efficacy in dependent than nondependent persons, especially for those forms of treatment that are associated with low levels of compliance. As Balint (1964) and others (e.g., Crowder, 1972; Dollard & Miller, 1950) have noted, dependency can—if handled correctly by the therapist—be an important contributor to the development and maintenance of a good "working alliance" between patient and therapist.

Along slightly different lines, it is noteworthy that one dependency-related issue that has received a tremendous amount of attention from clinicians in recent years has received virtually no attention from clinical researchers. As psychologists, psychiatrists, and other mental health professionals have come to recognize the myriad ways that addictive disorders affect the substance-abusing individual's family, friends, and coworkers, the term *co-dependency* has become increasingly popular within the therapeutic community. Morgan (1991) summarized the various definitions of co-dependency that have been employed by clinicians in recent years. These definitions make clear that there are some important parallels between the emerging concept of co-dependency and the more well-established concept of the dependent personality. Perusal of one recent clinical definition of co-dependency illustrates these parallels: Wegscheider-Cruse (1985) defined co-dependency as a syndrome characterized by "preoccupation and extreme dependency (emotional, social and sometimes physical) on a person or object. Eventually, this dependence on another person becomes a pathological condition that affects the co-dependent [individual] in all of her relationships" (p. 2).

While there are some noteworthy parallels between the concepts of dependency and co-dependency, there are also some critical differences between these two constructs (e.g., Lyon & Greenberg, 1991; Morgan, 1991; O'Brien & Gaborit, 1992; O'Gorman, 1991). Dependency and co-dependency are qualitatively different—albeit related—phenomena. In this context, a number of important questions regarding the relationship of these two constructs remain unanswered. For example, the degree to which an individual with a dependent personality orientation is at increased risk for pathological co-dependency is an empirical question that has not yet been addressed. Conversely, the degree to which involvement in a co-dependent relationship produces increases in a person's dependent behavior in other relationships remains open to question. Despite the fact that Wegscheider-Cruse (1985) and others (e.g., Rathbone-McCuan, Dyer, & Wartman, 1991) assert that co-dependent behavior generalizes to other interpersonal relationships, there are no data available that address this question directly. Exploring the relationship between the constructs of dependency and co-dependency will be an important task for clinical researchers during the coming years.

Although the most obvious applications of dependency research involve psychological and medical treatment, it is also worthwhile to consider some of the potential applications of dependency research in nonclinical settings. Several possibilities present themselves in this context. First, the results of numerous studies suggest that dependency might predict important aspects of behavior in academic settings (see, for example, research on dependency and help seeking, suggestibility, compliance, creativity, performance anxiety, sociometric status, and school phobias). Unfortunately, as noted in Chapter 4, there have been very few studies examining directly the dependency–academic performance relationship. However, the most well-designed investigation of this issue found that dependency was associated with scholastic underachievement (Tesser & Blusiewicz, 1987). By identifying children who show elevated levels of dependent behavior in preschool and kindergarten, school officials might be able to identify children who are at risk for subsequent academic (and social) difficulties.

Along different lines, there is some evidence that dependency plays a role in predicting individuals' attitudes toward certain social service (i.e., welfare and disability) programs. In an early study in this area, Pruitt and Vandecastle (1962) found that level of dependency predicted welfare chronicity in a sample of 30 community subjects, with dependent welfare recipients (selected according to scores on Navran's [1954] MMPI Dy scale) remaining on welfare for a significantly longer period than nondependent welfare recipients. These results parallel Greenberg and Bornstein's (1989) findings (discussed earlier), which indicated that dependent psychiatric patients remain in the hospital significantly longer than do nondependent psychiatric patients.

Although Pruitt and Vandecastle's (1962) findings suggest that high levels of dependency are associated with increased reliance on welfare, Kilbourne and Kilbourne (1983) subsequently found that the experience of receiving welfare and disability payments can—in and of itself—result in increases in dependent feelings and behaviors. Kilbourne and Kilbourne's results are consistent with findings regarding "institutional dependency" that were discussed in Chapters 7, 8, and 9: Just as hospitalization can induce dependent attitudes and behaviors in medical and psychiatric patients, receiving welfare or disability payments can induce dependent attitudes and behaviors in individuals who participate in these social service programs.

Aside from possible applications of dependency research in clinical, academic, and social service settings, it appears that dependency can predict important aspects of an individual's behavior in structured and unstructured group decision-making situations. If, as the studies discussed in Chapter 4 suggest, dependency is associated with suggestibility, compliance, and interpersonal yielding, then it is likely that dependency will be an important predictor of an individual's behavior in various types of problem-solving groups (e.g., juries, committees, other task-oriented work groups). Research confirms that in a wide variety of group decision-making situations, the behavior of individuals is strongly influenced by implicit or explicit pressure to conform to the majority opinion (see Aronson, 1992; Goethals & Zanna, 1979). Such conformity pressures are likely to be particularly salient for the dependent person.

Dependency also has important implications for understanding and predicting the behavior exhibited by subjects in psychology experiments. Studies have demonstrated that (1) certain personality characteristics influence college students' willingness to participate in psychology experiments (Jackson, Procidano, & Cohen, 1989); (2) subjects who participate in experiments at different times during the semester differ on various personality dimensions (Holden & Reddon, 1987); and (3) subjects' personality traits affect their behavior during psychology experiments in important ways (Rosenthal & Rosnow, 1975). The studies reviewed in Chapter 4 confirm that dependency plays a role in all three of these areas (see, e.g., Bornstein & Masling, 1985; Masling et al., 1981; Shilkret & Masling, 1981; Weiss, 1969).

In general, it seems that dependent individuals make good experimental subjects: They sign up for psychology experiments when asked and comply with the perceived expectations of the experimenter during the experiment itself. Of course, it would not be feasible (or desirable) for experimenters to prescreen all potential subjects for level of dependency, selecting only highly dependent subjects for their experiments. However, the findings reported by Masling et al. (1981) and Bornstein and Masling (1985) suggest that experimenters need not take such elaborate precautions. These studies demonstrated that dependent subjects participate in psychology experiments earlier in the semester than do nondependent subjects. Thus, experimenters can "select" dependent (or nondependent) subjects for their experiments simply by running subjects at different times during the semester. Although this may not always be possible, the results of Masling et al.'s (1981) and Bornstein and Masling's (1985) investigations nonetheless suggest that experimenters can estimate the overall level of dependency in their subject sample simply by noting the time in the semester at which the subjects were run.

In closing, it is worthwhile to mention one possible application of developmental research on dependency. The findings discussed in this book have important implications for parenting practices. Specifically, the studies reviewed in Chapter 3 indicate that parenting practices that discourage independent decision making and autonomous behavior in young children can lead to high levels of dependency later in life. It goes without saying that parents have very different values, aspirations, and goals for their children. Some parents might believe that cooperativeness and compliance are more valuable traits than are independence and autonomy. Nonetheless, to the extent that parents are made aware of the links between overprotective, authoritarian parenting and the development of dependent personality traits in children, they can at least make an informed choice regarding their parenting practices in these areas.

## A FINAL COMMENT

Nearly 50 years ago, Sullivan (1947) described dependent individuals as "obedient children of a dominating parent. They go through life needing a strong person to make decisions for them. [They] learned their helplessness and clinging vine adaptation from parental example" (p. 84). Horney (1945) similarly argued that the dependent individual "has a pervasive feeling that he is weak and helpless. . . . His self-esteem rises and falls with [others'] approval and disapproval, their affection or lack of it" (pp. 52–56). The results of the studies reviewed in this book indicate that Sullivan's and Horney's views were remarkably prescient: Several decades of research confirm that the traits and behaviors attributed by these theoreticians to the dependent individual are in fact characteristic of dependent persons.

However, if there is one theme that I have tried to stress throughout this volume, it is that the traditional "deficit" view of dependency described by Sullivan (1947), Horney (1945), and others is overly narrow and unnecessarily pessimistic. Dependency has proven to be associated with positive as well as negative qualities. Thus, in addition to investigating the cognitive and attributional correlates of dependency; the interaction of dependency with situational demands, constraints, and expectations; and the practical implications of dependency research, investigators should now begin to devote more attention to examining the positive, adaptive qualities of dependent personality traits.

## NOTES

1. Millon (1981) has offered some interesting hypotheses in this area, arguing that "a gentle but fearful infant is likely to evoke warmth and overprotectiveness from a concerned mother. Such children invite excessive care from others, which may result in their learning to be overly dependent and comfortable with caretakers" (p. 124). Millon went on to speculate regarding some possible neurological and physiochemical patterns that might underlie (or result from) dependency-related differences in temperament. He suggested: "[R]eticular arousal mechanisms may be sluggish in these individuals, giving rise to deficient coping under conditions of stress. At the same time, they may be overly endowed in limbic regions associated with fear, pain and sadness. . . . Such individuals may experience intense emotional turmoil but lack the sustained adrenal reaction necessary for effective coping responses" (p. 125).

Although Millon's hypotheses regarding the neurological underpinnings of dependency remain untested, they provide a useful starting point for researchers interested in examining the possibility that dependent personality traits may be traced in part to individual differences in neurophysiological structure and function.

2. Bowlby (1969, 1973, 1980) and others (e.g., Main et al., 1985) refer to these internalized mental representations of the self and others as "working models" of self–other interactions (see Greenberg & Mitchell [1983] for a detailed discussion of the various terms used by object relations and attachment theorists to describe mental representations of significant figures).

3. The notion that separate "active" and "passive" manifestations of dependency exist has been discussed elsewhere (e.g., Abraham, 1927; Gewirtz, 1956a;

Levy, 1943). However, these earlier theorists and researchers typically conceptualized "active" and "passive" dependency as separate personality dimensions, arguing that some individuals are characterized by an active-dependent personality style while other individuals are characterized by a passive-dependent personality style. I am suggesting that dependent individuals show *both* active and passive dependency-related behaviors, with the nature of the behavior that is exhibited in a given situation determined largely by the demands and contraints of that situation.

4. It is worth noting, parenthetically, that the motivational, cognitive, and affective components of dependency depicted in this model can, in a relatively straightforward way, account for certain of the findings discussed in earlier chapters. For example, it is clear that the increased rates of school phobia and agoraphobia that are found in dependent individuals reflect in part the dependent person's desire to maintain close ties to protecting, nurturing figures. Similarly, the affective component of dependency may well account for Tesser and Blusiewicz's (1987) finding that dependency is associated with scholastic underachievement: To the extent that dependency is associated with fear of evaluation by figures of authority, academic performance is likely to suffer. Finally, the motivational, affective, and behavioral components of dependency may all be implicated in the acquisition of the dysfunctional defensive style discussed by Bornstein et al. (1990) and Levit (1991), wherein the dependent person turns anger and aggression inward rather than expressing these "negative" emotions directly.

# References

Abraham, K. (1927). The influence of oral erotism on character formation. In C. A. D. Bryan & A. Strachey (Eds.), *Selected papers on psycho-analysis* (pp. 393–406). London: Hogarth Press.

Abramson, L., Seligman, M. E. P., & Teasdale, J. (1978). Learned helplessness in humans: Critique and reformulation. *Journal of Abnormal Psychology, 87*, 49–74.

Adler, D. A., Drake, R. E., & Teague, G. B. (1990). Clinicians' practices in personality assessment: Does gender influence the use of DSM-III Axis II? *Comprehensive Psychiatry, 31*, 125–133.

Agoustinos, M. (1986). Psychiatric inpatients' attitudes toward mental disorder and tendency to adopt a sick role. *Psychological Reports, 58*, 495–498.

Agrawal, K., & Rai, S. N. (1988). Post-noise frustration tolerance as a function of controllability of noise and dependence proneness. *Indian Journal of Psychometry and Education, 19*, 85–89.

Ainsworth, M. D. S. (1969). Object relations, dependency and attachment: A theoretical review of the infant–mother relationship. *Child Development, 40*, 969–1025.

Ainsworth, M. D. S. (1972). Attachment and dependency: A comparison. In J. L. Gewirtz (Ed.), *Attachment and dependency* (pp. 97–137). New York: Wiley.

Ainsworth, M. D. S. (1989). Attachments beyond infancy. *American Psychologist, 44*, 709–716.

Akiskal, H. S., Hirschfeld, R. M. A., & Yerevanian, B. I. (1983). The relationship of personality to affective disorders. *Archives of General Psychiatry, 40*, 801–810.

Alam, K. (1986). An experimental study of retention in relation to approval motive and dependence proneness. *Journal of Psychological Research, 30*, 144–149.

Alam, K., Khan, M. I., & Khan, S. A. (1986). Effect of approval motive and dependence proneness on retention: An experimental study. *Perspectives in Psychological Research, 9*, 32–36.

Alexander, F. (1950). *Psychosomatic medicine*. New York: W. W. Norton.

Alexander, F., French, T. M., & Pollock, G. H. (1968). *Psychosomatic specificity*. Chicago: University of Chicago Press.

Alexander, J. (1970). On dependence and independence. *Bulletin of the Philadelphia Association for Psychoanalysis, 20*, 49–57.

Almgren, P. E., Nordgren, L., & Skantze, H. (1978). A retrospective study of operationally defined hysterics. *British Journal of Psychiatry, 132,* 67–73.

Alnaes, R., & Torgerson, S. (1988a). DSM-III symptom disorders (Axis I) and personality disorders (Axis II) in an outpatient population. *Acta Psychiatrica Scandinavica, 78,* 348–355.

Alnaes, R., & Torgerson, S. (1988b). The relationship between DSM-III symptom disorders (Axis I) and personality disorders (Axis II) in an outpatient population. *Acta Psychiatrica Scandinavica, 78,* 485–492.

Alnaes, R., & Torgerson, S. (1990). DSM-III personality disorders among patients with major depression, anxiety disorders and mixed conditions. *Journal of Nervous and Mental Disease, 178,* 693–698.

Alsop, A. E. (1984). Purley Day Hospital: An appraisal with special reference to institutionalized behavior and dependence. *Occupational Therapy, 47,* 306–310.

American Psychiatric Association. (1952). *Diagnostic and statistical manual of mental disorders* (1st ed.). Washington, DC: Author.

American Psychiatric Association. (1968). *Diagnostic and statistical manual of mental disorders* (2nd ed.). Washington, DC: Author.

American Psychiatric Association. (1980). *Diagnostic and statistical manual of mental disorders* (3rd ed.). Washington, DC: Author.

American Psychiatric Association. (1987). *Diagnostic and statistical manual of mental disorders* (3rd ed., rev.). Washington, DC: Author.

American Psychiatric Association. (1991). *DSM-IV options book.* Washington, DC: Author.

Ammon, G. (1979). *Psychoanalysis and psychosomatics.* New York: Springer-Verlag.

Anderson, K. L. (1986). Androgeny, flexibility and individualism. *Journal of Personality Assessment, 50,* 265–278.

Andrews, B., & Brown, G. W. (1988). Social support, onset of depression and personality. *Social Psychiatry and Psychiatric Epidemiology, 23,* 99–108.

Antoni, M., Levine, J., Tischer, P., Green, C., & Millon, T. (1987). Refining personality assessments by combining MCMI high-point profiles and MMPI codes, Part V: MMPI code 78/87. *Journal of Personality Assessment, 51,* 375–387.

Aronson, E. (1992). *The social animal.* New York: W. H. Freeman.

Aronson, M. L. (1953). A study of the Freudian theory of paranoia by means of the Blacky pictures. *Journal of Projective Techniques, 17,* 3–19.

Asch, S. E. (1956). Studies of independence and conformity: A minority of one against a unanimous majority. *Psychological Monographs, 70* (9, Whole No. 416).

Ashmore, R. D. (1981). Sex stereotypes and implicit personality theory. In D. L. Hamilton (Ed.), *Cognitive processes in stereotyping and intergroup behavior* (pp. 37–81). Hillsdale, NJ: Erlbaum.

Assor, A., Aronoff, J., & Messe, L. (1981). Attribute relevance as a moderator of the effects of motivation on impression formation. *Journal of Personality and Social Psychology, 41,* 789–796.

Bacon, M. K., Barry, H., & Child, I. L. (1965). A cross-cultural study of drinking: Relations to other features of culture. *Quarterly Journal of Studies on Alcohol,* Suppl. 3, 29–48.

Bahnson, C. B. (1975). Emotional and personality characteristics of patients. In A. Sardnick (Ed.), *Recent developments in medical oncology* (pp. 91–117). Baltimore, MD: University Park Press.

Bahnson, C. B., & Bahnson, M. B. (1964a). Denial and repression of primitive impulses and of disturbing emotions in patients with malignant neoplasms. In D. M. Kissel & L. L. LeShan (Eds.), *Psychosomatic aspects of neoplastic disease* (pp. 42–62). Philadelphia: Lippincott.

Bahnson, C. B., & Bahnson, M. B. (1964b). Cancer as an alternative to psychosis. In D. M. Kissel & L. L. LeShan (Eds.), *Psychosomatic aspects of neoplastic disease* (pp. 184–202). Philadelphia: Lippincott.

Bahnson, C. B., & Bahnson, M. B. (1966). Role of ego defenses: Denial and repression in the etiology of malignant neoplasm. *Annals of the New York Academy of Sciences, 125,* 827–845.

Baker, L. D., & Reitz, H. J. (1978). Altruism toward the blind: Effects of sex of helper and dependency of victim. *Journal of Social Psychology, 104,* 19–28.

Bales, R. F. (1970). *Personality and interpersonal behavior.* New York: Holt, Rinehart & Winston.

Balint, M. (1964). *The doctor, his patient and the illness.* London: Pitman Medical.

Bandura, A. (1977). Self-efficacy: Toward a unifying theory of behavior change. *Psychological Review, 84,* 191–215.

Bandura, A., & Walters, R. H. (1959). *Adolescent aggression.* New York: Ronald.

Bandura, A., & Walters, R. H. (1963). *Social learning and personality development.* New York: Holt, Rinehart & Winston.

Banu, S., & Puhan, B. N. (1983). Social responsibility and dependence proneness in Indian and Bangladeshi men and women. *Personality Study and Group Behavior, 3,* 1–5.

Barnes, R. D., Ickes, W., & Kidd, R. F. (1979). Effects of the perceived intentionality and stability of another's dependency on helping behavior. *Personality and Social Psychology Bulletin, 5,* 367–372.

Barry, H., Barry, H., & Lindemann, E. (1965). Dependency in adult patients following early maternal bereavement. *Journal of Nervous and Mental Disease, 140,* 196–206.

Bartholomew, K., & Horowitz, L. M. (1991). Attachment styles among young adults. *Journal of Personality and Social Psychology, 61,* 226–244.

Barton, E. M., Baltes, M. M., & Orzech, M. J. (1980). Etiology of dependence in older nursing home residents during morning care: The role of staff behavior. *Journal of Personality and Social Psychology, 38,* 423–431.

Bartrop, R. W., Luckhurst, E., Lazarus, L., Kiloh, L. G., & Penny, R. (1977). Depressed lymphocyte function after bereavement. *The Lancet, 1,* 834–836.

Bateson, G., Jackson, D. D., Haley, J., & Weakland, J. (1956). Toward a theory of schizophrenia. *Behavioral Science, 1,* 251–264.

Battistich, V. A., & Aronoff, J. (1985). Perceiver, target and situational influences on social cognition. *Journal of Personality and Social Psychology, 49,* 788–798.

Bauermeister, M. (1982). Dependence. *International Journal of Offender Therapy and Comparative Criminology, 26,* 138–144.

Baumrind, D. (1967). Child care practices anteceding three patterns of preschool behavior. *Genetic Psychology Monographs*, *75*, 43–88.

Baumrind, D. (1971). Current patterns of parental authority. *Developmental Psychology Monograph*, *4* (1, Pt. 2), 1–173.

Baumrind, D. (1973). The development of instrumental competence through socialization. In A. D. Pick (Ed.), *Minnesota symposium on child psychology* (Vol. 7, pp. 3–46). Minneapolis, MN: University of Minnesota Press.

Baumrind, D. (1980). New directions in socialization research. *American Psychologist*, *35*, 639–652.

Baumrind, D., & Black, A. E. (1967). Socialization practices associated with dimensions of competence in preschool boys and girls. *Child Development*, *38*, 291–327.

Beall, C. M., & Goldstein, M. C. (1982). Work, aging and dependency in a Sherpa population in Nepal. *Social Science and Medicine*, *16*, 141– 147.

Beck, A. T. (1967). *Depression: Clinical, experimental and theoretical aspects.* New York: Holber.

Beck, A. T., Epstein, N., Harrison, R. P., & Emery, G. (1983). *Development of the Sociotropy–Autonomy Scale: A measure of personality factors in psychopathology.* Unpublished manuscript.

Becker, W. C., Peterson, D. R., Luria, Z., Shoemaker, D. J., & Hellmer, L. A. (1962). Relations of factors derived from parent interview ratings to behavior problems of five year olds. *Child Development*, *33*, 509–535.

Beckwith, J. B. (1986). Eating, drinking and smoking and their relationship in adult women. *Psychological Reports*, *59*, 1095–1089.

Beebe, B. (1986). Mother–infant mutual influence and precursors of self and object representations. In J. Masling (Ed.), *Empirical studies of psychoanalytic theories* (Vol. 2, pp. 27–48). Hillsdale, NJ: Erlbaum.

Beller, E. K. (1955). Dependency and independence in young children. *Journal of Genetic Psychology*, *87*, 23–25.

Beller, E. K. (1957). Dependency and autonomous achievement-striving related to orality and anality in early childhood. *Child Development*, *29*, 287–315.

Beller, E. K. (1959). Exploratory studies of dependency. *Transactions of the New York Academy of Sciences*, *21*, 414–426.

Bem, S. (1974). The measurement of psychological androgeny. *Journal of Consulting and Clinical Psychology*, *42*, 155–162.

Benfari, R. C. (1969). Relationship between early dependence training and the patient-therapist dyad. *Psychological Reports*, *25*, 552–554.

Bennie, E. H., & Sclare, A. B. (1969). The battered child syndrome. *American Journal of Psychiatry*, *125*, 975–979.

Berg, I. (1974). A self-administered dependency questionnaire for use with mothers of schoolchildren. *British Journal of Psychiatry*, *124*, 1–9.

Berg, I., & McGuire, R. (1974). Are mothers of school-phobic adolescents overprotective? *British Journal of Psychiatry*, *124*, 10–13.

Berg, I., McGuire, R., & Whelan, E. (1973). The Highlands Dependency Questionnaire. *Journal of Child Psychology and Psychiatry*, *14*, 107–124.

Berg, I., Nichols, K., & Pritchard, C. (1969). School phobia: Its classification and relationship to dependency. *Journal of Child Psychology and Psychiatry, 10,* 123–141.

Berger, L. (1959). Cross-validation of primary and reactive personality patterns with non-ulcer surgical patients. *Journal of Projective Techniques, 23,* 8–11.

Berkowitz, L. (1969). Resistance to improper dependency relationships. *Journal of Experimental Social Psychology, 5,* 283–294.

Berkowitz, L. (1970). The self, selfishness and altruism. In J. Macauley & L. Berkowitz (Eds.), *Altruism and helping behavior* (pp. 143–151). New York: Academic Press.

Berkowitz, L. (1972). Social norms, feelings, and other factors affecting helping and altruism. In L. Berkowitz (Ed.), *Advances in experimental social psychology* (Vol. 6, pp. 63–108). New York: Academic Press.

Berkowitz, L., & Connor, W. H. (1966). Success, failure and social responsibility. *Journal of Personality and Social Psychology, 4,* 664–669.

Berkowitz, L., & Daniels, L. R. (1963). Responsibility and dependency. *Journal of Abnormal and Social Psychology, 66,* 429–436.

Berkowitz, L., & Daniels, L. R. (1964). Affecting the salience of the social responsibility norm: Effects of past help on the response to dependency relationships. *Journal of Abnormal and Social Psychology, 68,* 275–281.

Berkowitz, L., Klanderman, S. B., & Harris, R. (1964). Effects of experimenter awareness and sex of subject and experimenter on reactions to dependency relationships. *Sociometry, 27,* 327–337.

Bernardin, A., & Jessor, R. (1957). A construct validation of the Edwards Personal Preference Schedule with respect to dependency. *Journal of Consulting Psychology, 21,* 63–67.

Berry, C. M. (1986). Dependent personality disorder: Case conference. *Journal of Psychiatry and Christianity, 4,* 42–47.

Berscheid, E., & Fei, J. (1977). Romantic love and sexual jealousy. In G. Clanton & L. G. Smith (Eds.), *Jealousy* (pp. 101–109). Englewood Cliffs, NJ: Prentice-Hall.

Bertrand, S., & Masling, J. (1969). Oral imagery and alcoholism. *Journal of Abnormal Psychology, 74,* 50–53.

Beswick, D. G., & Cox, F. N. (1958). Reputed aggression and dependence in children. *Australian Journal of Psychology, 10,* 144–150.

Bhogle, S. (1983). Antecedents of dependency behavior in children of low social class. *Psychological Studies, 28,* 92–95.

Biaggio, M. K., Godwin, W. H., & Baldwin, H. K. (1984). Response to interpersonal request styles by dependent and overcontrolled–hostile personalities. *Journal of Clinical Psychology, 40,* 833–836.

Bird, H. W., Martin, P. A., & Schuham, A. (1983). The marriage of the "collapsible" man of prominence. *American Journal of Psychiatry, 140,* 290–295.

Birtchnell, J. (1980). Women whose mothers died in childhood: An outcome study. *Psychological Medicine, 10,* 699–713.

Birtchnell, J. (1984). Dependence and its relationship to depression. *British Journal of Medical Psychology, 57,* 215–225.

Birtchnell, J. (1987). Attachment–detachment, directiveness–receptiveness: A system for classifying interpersonal attitudes and behavior. *British Journal of Medical Psychology*, *60*, 17–27.

Birtchnell, J. (1988a). Defining dependence. *British Journal of Medical Psychology*, *61*, 111–123.

Birtchnell, J. (1988b). The assessment of the marital relationship by questionnaire. *Sexual and Marital Therapy*, *3*, 57–70.

Birtchnell, J. (1991a). Redefining dependence: A reply to Cadbury's critique. *British Journal of Medical Psychology*, *64*, 253–261.

Birtchnell, J. (1991b). The measurement of dependence by questionnaire. *Journal of Personality Disorders*, *5*, 281–295.

Birtchnell, J., & Kennard, J. (1983). What does the MMPI dependency scale really measure? *Journal of Clinical Psychology*, *39*, 532–543.

Black, D. W., Goldstein, R. B., & Mason, E. E. (1992). Prevalence of mental disorder in 88 morbidly obese bariatric clinic patients. *American Journal of Psychiatry*, *149*, 227–234.

Blane, H. T., & Chafetz, M. E. (1971). Dependency conflict and sex-role identity in drinking delinquents. *Quarterly Journal of Studies on Alcohol*, *32*, 1025–1039.

Blaney, P. H., & Kutcher, G. S. (1991). Measures of depressive dimensions: Are they interchangeable? *Journal of Personality Assessment*, *56*, 502–512.

Blashfield, R. K., & Livesley, W. J. (1991). Metaphorical analysis of psychiatric classification as a psychological test. *Journal of Abnormal Psychology*, *100*, 262–270.

Blatt, S. J. (1974). Levels of object representation in anaclitic and introjective depression. *Psychoanalytic Study of the Child*, *29*, 107–157.

Blatt, S. J., Allison, J., & Feirstein, A. (1969). The capacity to cope with cognitive complexity. *Journal of Personality*, *37*, 269–288.

Blatt, S. J., D'Afflitti, J. P., & Quinlan, D. M. (1976). Experiences of depression in normal young adults. *Journal of Abnormal Psychology*, *85*, 383–389.

Blatt, S. J., & Homann, E. (1992). Parent–child interaction in the etiology of dependent and self-critical depression. *Clinical Psychology Review*, *12*, 47–91.

Blatt, S. J., Quinlan, D. M., Chevron, E. S., McDonald, C., & Zuroff, D. (1982). Dependency and self-criticism: Psychological dimensions of depression. *Journal of Consulting and Clinical Psychology*, *50*, 113–124.

Blatt, S. J., Rounsaville, B., Eyre, S. L., & Wilber, C. (1984). The psychodynamics of opiate addiction. *Journal of Nervous and Mental Disease*, *172*, 342–352.

Blatt, S. J., Wein, S. J., Chevron, E. S., & Quinlan, D. M. (1979). Parental representations and depression in normal young adults. *Journal of Abnormal Psychology*, *88*, 388–397.

Block, J. (1971). *Lives through time*. Berkeley, CA: Bancroft Books.

Block, J., Block, J. L., & Keyes, S. (1988). Longitudinally foretelling drug usage in adolescence: Early childhood and environmental precursors. *Child Development*, *59*, 336–355.

Bloom, L. (1982). Socialization and dependence in Nigeria. *Journal of Social Psychology*, *117*, 3–12.

Blum, G. S. (1949). A study of the psychoanalytic theory of psychosexual development. *Genetic Psychology Monographs*, *39*, 3–99.

Blum, G. S., & Miller, D. (1952). Exploring the psychoanalytic theory of the "oral character." *Journal of Personality*, *20*, 287–304.

Boehm, L. (1947). The development of independence: A comparative study. *Child Development*, *28*, 85–92.

Booth, T. (1986). Institutional regimes and induced dependency in homes for the aged. *The Gerontologist*, *26*, 418–423.

Bornstein, R. F. (1992). The dependent personality: Developmental, social and clinical perspectives. *Psychological Bulletin*, *112*, 3–23.

Bornstein, R. F., Galley, D. J., & Leone, D. R. (1986). Parental representations and orality. *Journal of Personality Assessment*, *50*, 80–89.

Bornstein, R. F., & Greenberg, R. P. (1991). Dependency and eating disorders in female psychiatric inpatients. *Journal of Nervous and Mental Disease*, *179*, 148–152.

Bornstein, R. F., Greenberg, R. P., Leone, D. R., & Galley, D. J. (1990). Defense mechanism correlates of orality. *Journal of the American Academy of Psychoanalysis*, *18*, 654–666.

Bornstein, R. F., & Johnson, J. G. (1990). Dependency and psychopathology in a nonclinical sample. *Journal of Social Behavior and Personality*, *5*, 417–422.

Bornstein, R. F., Leone, D. R., & Galley, D. J. (1988a). Rorschach measures of oral dependence and the internalized self-representation in normal college students. *Journal of Personality Assessment*, *52*, 648–657.

Bornstein, R. F., & Masling, J. M. (1985). Orality and latency of volunteering to serve as experimental subjects: A replication. *Journal of Personality Assessment*, *49*, 306–310.

Bornstein, R. F., Masling, J. M., & Poynton, F. G. (1987). Orality as a factor in interpersonal yielding. *Psychoanalytic Psychology*, *4*, 161–170.

Bornstein, R. F., O'Neill, R. M., Galley, D. J., Leone, D. R., & Castrianno, L. M. (1988b). Body image aberration and orality. *Journal of Personality Disorders*, *2*, 315–322.

Bornstein, R. F., Poynton, F. G., & Masling, J. M. (1985). Orality and depression: An empirical study. *Psychoanalytic Psychology*, *2*, 241–249.

Boss, M. (1977). *Existential foundations of medicine and psychology*. New York: Jason Aronson.

Bowlby, J. (1953). Some pathological processes set in place by early mother–child separation. *Journal of Mental Science*, *99*, 265–272.

Bowlby, J. (1969). *Attachment*. New York: Basic Books.

Bowlby, J. (1973). *Separation: Anxiety and anger*. New York: Basic Books.

Bowlby, J. (1980). *Loss: Sadness and depression*. New York: Basic Books.

Brewin, C. R., & Furnham, A. (1987). Dependency, self-criticism and depressive attributional style. *British Journal of Clinical Psychology*, *26*, 225–226.

Broverman, I., Vogel, S., Broverman, D., Clarkson, F. E., & Rosenkrantz, P. S. (1972). Sex-role stereotypes: A current appraisal. *Journal of Social Issues*, *28*, 59–78.

Brown, J. S., & Rawlinson, M. (1975). Relinquishing the sick role following open heart surgery. *Journal of Health and Social Behavior*, *16*, 12–27.

Brown, J. D., & Silberschatz, G. (1989). Dependency, self-criticism and depressive attributional style. *Journal of Abnormal Psychology*, *98*, 187–188.

Bruch, H. (1973). *Eating disorders: Anorexia, bulimia and the person within*. New York: Basic Books.

Buglass, D., Clarke, J., Henderson, A. S., Kreitman, N., & Presley, A. S. (1977). A study of agoraphobic housewives. *Psychological Medicine*, *7*, 73–86.

Burton, A., McGregor, H., & Berry, P. (1979). The effects of social reinforcement on dominant and dependent mildly intellectually handicapped school-leavers. *British Journal of Social and Clinical Psychology*, *18*, 129–133.

Bush, C. R., Bush, J. P., & Jennings, J. (1988). Effects of jealousy threats on relationship perceptions and emotions. *Journal of Social and Personal Relationships*, *5*, 285–303.

Buss, A. H., & Plomin, R. (1984). *Temperament: Early developing personality traits*. Hillsdale, NJ: Erlbaum.

Buss, D. M. (1983). Evolutionary biology and personality psychology: Implications of genetic variability. *Personality and Individual Differences*, *4*, 51–63.

Button, A. D. (1956). A study of alcoholics on the MMPI. *Quarterly Journal of Studies on Alcohol*, *17*, 263–281.

Buunk, B. (1982). Anticipated sexual jealousy: Its relationship to self-esteem, dependency and reciprocity. *Personality and Social Psychology Bulletin*, *8*, 310–316.

Buunk, B. (1983). The role of attributions and dependency in jealousy. *Nederlands Tijdschrift voor Psychologie*, *38*, 301–311.

Cacioppo, J. T., & Petty, R. E. (1982). The need for cognition. *Journal of Personality and Social Psychology*, *42*, 116–131.

Cadbury, S. (1991). The concept of dependence as developed by Birtchnell: A critical evaluation. *British Journal of Medical Psychology*, *64*, 237–251.

Cairns, R. B. (1961). The influence of dependency inhibition on the effectiveness of social reinforcement. *Journal of Personality*, *29*, 466–488.

Cairns, R. B. (1972). Attachment and dependency: A psychobiological and social learning synthesis. In J. L. Gewirtz (Ed.), *Attachment and dependency* (pp. 179–216). New York: Wiley.

Cairns, R. B., & Lewis, M. (1962). Dependency and the reinforcement value of a verbal stimulus. *Journal of Consulting Psychology*, *26*, 1–8.

Calsyn, D. A., & Saxon, A. J. (1990). Personality disorder subtypes among cocaine and opioid addicts using the MCMI. *International Journal of the Addictions*, *25*, 1037–1049.

Calsyn, D. A., Saxon, A. J., & Daisy, F. (1991). Validity of the MCMI drug abuse scale varies as a function of drug choice, race, and Axis II subtype. *American Journal of Drug and Alcohol Abuse*, *17*, 153–159.

Carnes, B. A. (1984). Concept analysis: Dependence. *Critical Care Quarterly*, *6*, 29–39.

Caspi, A., Bem, D. J., & Elder, G. H. (1989). Continuities and consequences of interactional styles across the life course. *Journal of Personality*, *57*, 375–406.

Cattell, R. B. (1966). *The scientific analysis of personality*. Chicago: Aldine.

Chadha, N. K. (1983). A study of dependence proneness and test anxiety in school-going children. *Indian Psychological Review*, *24*, 34–38.

Cherniss, C. (1972). Personality and ideology: A personological study of women's liberation. *Psychiatry*, *35*, 109–125.

Chesney, M. A., & Rosenman, R. H. (1985). *Anger and hostility in cardiovascular and behavioral disorders.* New York: Hemisphere.

Chevron, E. S., Quinlan, D. M., & Blatt, S. J. (1978). Sex roles and gender differences in the experience of depression. *Journal of Abnormal Psychology, 87,* 680–683.

Chiriboga, D. A., & Thurnher, M. (1980). Marital lifestyles and adjustment to separation. *Journal of Divorce, 3,* 379–390.

Cochrane, W. A. (1965). The battered child syndrome. *Canadian Journal of Public Health, 56,* 193–196.

Colgan, P. (1987). Treatment of dependency disorders in men: Toward a balance of identity and intimacy. *Journal of Chemical Dependency Treatment, 1,* 205–227.

Collins, N. J., & Read, S. J. (1990). Adult attachment, working models and relationship quality in dating couples. *Journal of Personality and Social Psychology, 58,* 644–663.

Colton, S. I. (1980). Instrumental dependency in institutionalized schizophrenics. *Psychosocial Rehabilitation Journal, 4,* 9–18.

Conley, J. J. (1980). Family configuration as an etiological factor in alcoholism. *Journal of Abnormal Psychology, 89,* 670–673.

Cooperman, M., & Child, I. (1971). Differential effects of positive and negative reinforcement on two psychoanalytic character types. *Journal of Consulting and Clinical Psychology, 37,* 57–59.

Corbisiero, J. R., & Reznikoff, M. (1991). The relationship between personality type and style of alcohol use. *Journal of Clinical Psychology, 47,* 291–298.

Couch, A., & Keniston, K. (1960). Yeasayers and naysayers: Agreeing response set as a personality variable. *Journal of Abnormal and Social Psychology, 60,* 151–174.

Craig, R. J. (1988). A psychometric study of the prevalence of DSM-III personality disorders among treated opiate addicts. *International Journal of the Addictions, 23,* 115–124.

Craig, R. J., Verinis, J. S., & Wexler, S. (1985). Personality characteristics of drug addicts and alcoholics on the MCMI. *Journal of Personality Assessment, 49,* 156–160.

Cramer, P., Blatt, S. J., & Ford, R. Q. (1988). Defense mechanisms in the anaclitic and introjective personality configuration. *Journal of Consulting and Clinical Psychology, 56,* 610–616.

Crandall, V. G., Preston, A., & Rabson, A. (1960). Maternal reactions and the development of independence and achievement behavior in young children. *Child Development, 31,* 243–251.

Crowder, J. E. (1972). Relationship between therapist and client interpersonal behaviors and psychotherapy outcome. *Journal of Counseling Psychology, 19,* 68–75.

Crowne, D. P., & Marlowe, D. (1964). *The approval motive.* New York: Wiley.

Daniels, L. R., & Berkowitz, L. (1963). Liking and response to dependency relationships. *Human Relations, 16,* 141–148.

Danzinger, K. (1960). Independence training and social class in Java, Indonesia. *Journal of Social Psychology, 51,* 65–74.

Davanloo, H. (1990). *Unlocking the unconscious*. New York: Wiley.

Davis, M. S., & Eichorn, R. L. (1963). Compliance with medical regimens. *Journal of Health and Human Behavior*, *4*, 240–249.

Dempewolff, J. A. (1974). Some correlates of feminism. *Psychological Reports*, *34*, 671–676.

Derogatis, L. R., Lipman, R. S., & Covi, L. (1973). SCL-90: An outpatient psychiatric rating scale. *Psychopharmacology Bulletin*, *9*, 13–28.

Devito, A. J., & Kubis, J. K. (1983). Actual and recalled test anxiety and flexibility, rigidity and self-control. *Journal of Clinical Psychology*, *39*, 970–975.

DeVos, G. (1952). A quantitative approach to affective symbolism in Rorschach responses. *Journal of Projective Techniques*, *16*, 133–150.

Diener, R. G. (1967). Prediction of dependent behavior in specified situations from psychological tests. *Psychological Reports*, *20*, 103–108.

Doi, T. (1973). *The anatomy of dependence*. Tokyo: Kodansha.

Dollard, J., & Miller, N. E. (1950). *Personality and psychotherapy*. New York: McGraw-Hill.

Drake, R. E., Adler, D. A., & Vaillant, G. E. (1988). Antecedents of personality disorders in a community sample of men. *Journal of Personality Disorders*, *2*, 60–68.

Dunnington, M. J. (1957). Behavioral differences of sociometric status groups in a nursery school. *Child Development*, *28*, 103–111.

Dweck, C. S., & Leggett, E. L. (1988). A social–cognitive approach to motivation and personality. *Psychological Review*, *95*, 256–273.

Dworkin, R. H., Burke, B. B., Maher, B. A., & Gottesman, I. I. (1976). A longitudinal study of the genetics of personality. *Journal of Personality and Social Psychology*, *34*, 510–518.

Eagly, A. H., & Crowley, M. (1986). Gender and helping behavior: A meta-analytic review of the social psychological literature. *Psychological Bulletin*, *100*, 283–308.

Eddington, C., Piper, J., Tanna, B., Hodkinson, H. M., & Salmon, P. (1990). Relationships between happiness, behavioural status and dependency on others in elderly patients. *British Journal of Clinical Psychology*, *29*, 43–50.

Ederer, E. (1988). Dysthymia, psychosocial dependency, and self-esteem in ten-year-old boys and girls. *Studia Psychologica*, *30*, 227–235.

Edwards, A. L. (1959). *Manual for the Edwards Personal Preference Schedule*. New York: Psychological Corporation.

Egeland, B., & Sroufe, L. A. (1981). Developmental sequelae of maltreatment in infancy. In R. Rizley & D. Cicchetti (Eds.), *New directions for child development* (pp. 77–92). San Francisco: Jossey-Bass.

Emery, G., & Lesher, E. (1982). Treatment of depression in older adults: Personality considerations. *Psychotherapy*, *19*, 500–505.

Emmerich, W. (1964). Continuity and stability in early social development. *Child Development*, *35*, 311–322.

Emmerich, W. (1966). Continuity and stability in early social development, II: Teachers' ratings. *Child Development*, *37*, 17–27.

Engel, G. L. (1967). The concept of psychosomatic disorder. *Journal of Psychosomatic Research*, *11*, 3–9.

Evans, R. G. (1984). MMPI dependency scale norms for alcoholics and psychiatric inpatients. *Journal of Clinical Psychology*, *40*, 345–346.

Exline, R. V., & Messick, D. (1967). The effects of dependency and social reinforcement upon visual behavior during an interview. *British Journal of Social and Clinical Psychology*, *6*, 256–266.

Feeney, J. A., & Noller, P. (1990). Attachment style as a predictor of adult romantic relationships. *Journal of Personality and Social Psychology*, *58*, 281–291.

Feldman, G. (1978). The only child as a separate entity: Differences between only females and other firstborn females. *Psychological Reports*, *42*, 107–110.

Fenichel, O. (1945). *The psychoanalytic theory of neurosis*. New York: W. W. Norton.

Finn, M. E. (1955). Study in suicidal attempts. *Journal of Nervous and Mental Disease*, *121*, 172–176.

Finney, J. C. (1961). Some maternal influences on children's personality and character. *Genetic Psychology Monographs*, *63*, 199–278.

Finney, J. C. (1965). Development of a new set of MMPI scales. *Psychological Reports*, *17*, 707–713.

Finney, J. C. (1966). Relations and meaning of the new MMPI scales. *Psychological Reports*, *18*, 459–470.

Fisher, J. M., & Fisher, S. (1975). Response to cigarette deprivation as a function of oral fantasy. *Journal of Personality Assessment*, *39*, 381–385.

Fisher, S. (1967). Projective methodologies. In P. Farnsworth, O. McNemar, & Q. McNemar (Eds.), *Annual review of psychology* (pp. 165–190). Palo Alto, CA: Annual Reviews.

Fisher, S. (1970). *Body experience in fantasy and behavior*. New York: Appleton-Century-Crofts.

Fisher, S., & Greenberg, R. P. (1985). *The scientific credibility of Freud's theories and therapy*. New York: Columbia University Press.

Fisher, S., & Osofsky, H. (1967). Sexual responsiveness in women: Psychological correlates. *Archives of General Psychiatry*, *17*, 214–226.

Fitzgerald, B. J. (1958). Some relationships among projective test, interview and sociometric measures of dependent behavior. *Journal of Abnormal and Social Psychology*, *56*, 199–203.

Flanders, N. A., Anderson, J. P., & Amidon, E. J. (1961). Measuring dependence proneness in the classroom. *Educational and Psychological Measurement*, *21*, 575–587.

Frances, A., & Widiger, T. A. (1987). A critical review of four DSM-III personality disorders. In G. L. Tischler (Ed.), *Diagnosis and classification in psychiatry* (pp. 269–289). New York: Cambridge University Press.

Frank, E., Kupfer, D. J., Jacob, M., & Jarrett, D. (1987). Personality features and response to acute treatment in recurrent depression. *Journal of Personality Disorders*, *1*, 14–26.

Frank, S. J., Avery, C. B., & Laman, M. S. (1988). Young adults' perceptions of their relationships with their parents: Individual differences in connectedness, competence and emotional autonomy. *Developmental Psychology*, *24*, 729–737.

Freedman, D. G. (1971). An evolutionary approach to research on the life cycle. *Human Development*, *14*, 87–99.

Freud, S. (1953). Three essays on the theory of sexuality. In J. Strachey (Ed. & Trans.), *The standard edition of the complete psychological works of Sigmund Freud* (Vol. 7, pp. 125–248). London: Hogarth Press. (Original work published 1905.)

Freud, S. (1955). Character and anal erotism. In J. Strachey (Ed. & Trans.), *The standard edition of the complete psychological works of Sigmund Freud* (Vol. 9, pp. 167–176). London: Hogarth Press. (Original work published 1908.)

Freud, S. (1964). An outline of psychoanalysis. In J. Strachey (Ed. & Trans.), *The standard edition of the complete psychological works of Sigmund Freud* (Vol. 23, pp. 125–248). London: Hogarth Press. (Original work published 1938.)

Friedman, H. S., & Booth-Kewley, S. (1987). The disease-prone personality: A meta-analytic review of the construct. *American Psychologist, 42*, 539–555.

Friedman, J. (1959). Weight problems and psychological factors. *Journal of Consulting Psychology, 23*, 524–527.

Fromm, E. (1947). *Man for himself.* New York: Rinehart.

Fu, V. R., Hinkle, D. E., & Hanna, M. A. K. (1986). A three-generation study of the development of individual dependency and family interdependence. *Genetic Psychology Monographs, 112*, 153–171.

Fu, V. R., Hinkle, D. E., Shoffner, S, Martin, S., Carter, E., Clark, A., Cully, P., Disney, G., Ercali., G, Glover, E., Kenney, M., Lewis, H., Moak, S., Stalling, S., & Wakefield, T. (1984). Maternal dependency and childrearing attitudes among mothers of adolescent females. *Adolescence, 19*, 795–804.

Fujihara, T., & Kurokawa, M. (1981). An empirical study of Amae (dependence) in interpersonal relations. *Japanese Journal of Experimental Social Psychology, 21*, 53–62.

Gayford, J. J. (1975). Wife battering: A preliminary survey of 100 cases. *British Medical Journal, 1*, 194–197.

Geersten, H. R., & Gray, R. M. (1970). Familistic orientation and inclination toward adopting the sick role. *Journal of Marriage and the Family, 32*, 638–646.

Geshuri, Y. (1975). Discriminative observational learning: Effects of observed reward and dependency. *Child Development, 46*, 550–554.

Gewirtz, J. L. (1956a). A factor-analysis of some attention-seeking behaviors of young children. *Child Development, 27*, 17–36.

Gewirtz, J. L. (1956b). A program of research on the dimensions and antecedents of emotional dependence. *Child Development, 27*, 205–221.

Gewirtz, J. L. (1972). *Attachment and dependency.* New York: Wiley.

Gilbert, L. A. (1987). Male and female emotional dependency and its implications for the therapist–client relationship. *Professional Psychology, 18*, 555–561.

Gleser, G. C., & Ihilevich, D. (1969). An objective instrument for measuring defense mechanisms. *Journal of Consulting and Clinical Psychology, 33*, 51–60.

Glover, E. (1925). Notes on oral character formation. *International Journal of Psycho-Analysis, 6*, 131–154.

Goethals, G. P., & Zanna, M. P. (1979). The role of social comparison in choice shifts. *Journal of Personality and Social Psychology, 37*, 1469–1476.

Goldberg, J. O., Segal, Z. V., Vella, D. D., & Shaw, B. F. (1989). Depressive personality: MCMI profiles of sociotropic and autonomous subtypes. *Journal of Personality Disorders, 3*, 193–198.

Goldman-Eisler, F. (1948). Breast-feeding and character formation. *Journal of Personality*, *17*, 83–103.

Goldman-Eisler, F. (1950). The etiology of the oral character in psychoanalytic theory. *Journal of Personality*, *19*, 189–196.

Goldman-Eisler, F. (1951). The problem of "orality" and its origin in early childhood. *Journal of Mental Science*, *97*, 765–782.

Goldstein, A. (1970). Case conference: Some aspects of agoraphobia. *Journal of Behavior Therapy and Experimental Psychiatry*, *1*, 305–313.

Goldstein, A., & Chambless, D. (1978). A reanalysis of agoraphobia. *Behavior Therapy*, *9*, 47–59.

Golightly, C., Nelson, D., & Johnson, J. (1970). Children's dependency scale. *Developmental Psychology*, *3*, 114–118.

Gordon, M., & Tegtemeyer, P. F. (1983). Oral dependent content in children's Rorschach protocols. *Perceptual and Motor Skills*, *57*, 1163–1168.

Gorton, D. A. (1975). Response to threats as a function of tasks and personality. *Journal of Behavioral Science*, *2*, 121–129.

Gottheil, E. (1965a). Conceptions of orality and anality. *Journal of Nervous and Mental Disease*, *141*, 155–160.

Gottheil, E. (1965b). An empirical analysis of orality and anality. *Journal of Nervous and Mental Disease*, *141*, 308–317.

Gottheil, E., & Stone, G. C. (1968). Factor analytic study of orality and anality. *Journal of Nervous and Mental Disease*, *146*, 1–17.

Gough, H. G. (1950). The F minus K dissimulation index for the MMPI. *Journal of Consulting Psychology*, *14*, 408–413.

Graves, P. L., Mead, L. A., & Pearson, T. A. (1986). The Rorschach interaction scale as a potential predictor of cancer. *Psychosomatic Medicine*, *48*, 549–563.

Greenberg, J. R., & Mitchell, S. J. (1983). *Object relations in psychoanalytic theory*. Cambridge, MA: Harvard University Press.

Greenberg, R. P., & Bornstein, R. F. (1988a). The dependent personality, I: Risk for physical disorders. *Journal of Personality Disorders*, *2*, 126–135.

Greenberg, R. P., & Bornstein, R. F. (1988b). The dependent personality, II: Risk for psychological disorders. *Journal of Personality Disorders*, *2*, 136–143.

Greenberg, R. P., & Bornstein, R. F. (1989). Length of psychiatric hospitalization and oral dependency. *Journal of Personality Disorders*, *3*, 199–204.

Greenberg, R. P., & Dattore, P. J. (1981). The relationship between dependency and the development of cancer. *Psychosomatic Medicine*, *43*, 35–43.

Greenberg, R. P., & Fisher, S. (1977). The relationship between willingness to adopt the sick role and attitudes toward women. *Journal of Chronic Disease*, *30*, 29–37.

Greene, W. A. (1954). Psychological factors and reticuloendothelial disease. *Psychosomatic Medicine*, *16*, 220–230.

Greene, W. A., Young, L., & Swisher, S. N. (1956). Psychological factors and reticuloendothelial disease, II: Observations on a group of women with lymphomas and leukemias. *Psychosomatic Medicine*, *18*, 284–303.

Griffith, C. E. (1991). Personality and gender as factors in interpersonal negotiation. *Journal of Social Behavior and Personality*, *6*, 915–928.

Gruder, C. L. (1974). Cost and dependency as determinants of helping and exploitation. *Journal of Conflict Resolution*, *18*, 473–485.

Gruder, C. L., & Cook, T. D. (1971). Sex, dependency and helping. *Journal of Personality and Social Psychology*, *19*, 290–294.

Gruder, C. L., Romer, D., & Korth, B. (1978). Dependency and fault as determinants of helping. *Journal of Experimental Social Psychology*, *14*, 227–235.

Hammen, C. (1991). Generation of stress in the course of unipolar depression. *Journal of Abnormal Psychology*, *100*, 555–561.

Hammen, C., Ellicott, A., & Gitlin, M. (1989a). Vulnerability to specific life events and prediction of course of disorder in unipolar depressed patients. *Canadian Journal of Behavioral Science*, *21*, 377–388.

Hammen, C. L., Ellicott, A., Gitlin, M., & Jamison, K. R. (1989b). Sociotropy/autonomy and vulnerability of specific life events in patients with unipolar depression and bipolar disorders. *Journal of Abnormal Psychology*, *98*, 154–160.

Hammen, C. L., Marks, T., Mayol, A., & DeMayo, R. (1985). Depressive self-schemas, life stress and vulnerability to depression. *Journal of Abnormal Psychology*, *94*, 308–319.

Hammerschlag, C. A., Fisher, S., DeCosse, J., & Kaplan, E. (1964). Breast symptoms and patient delay: Psychological variables involved. *Cancer*, *17*, 1480–1485.

Handler, L. (1989). Utilization approaches and psychodynamic psychotherapy in a case of hospital phobia: An integrated approach. *American Journal of Clinical Hypnosis*, *31*, 257–263.

Harlow, H. F. (1958). The nature of love. *American Psychologist*, *13*, 673–685.

Harris, M. B., & Ho, J. (1984). Effects of degree, locus and controllability of dependency and sex of subject on anticipated and actual helping. *Journal of Social Psychology*, *122*, 245–255.

Harris, M. B., & Klingbeil, D. R. (1976). The effects of ethnicity of subject and accent and dependency of confederate on aggressiveness and altruism. *Journal of Social Psychology*, *98*, 47–53.

Harris, M. B., & Meyer, F. (1973). Dependency, threat and helping. *Journal of Social Psychology*, *90*, 239–242.

Harris, M. C. (1956). A study of behavior patterns in asthmatic children. *Journal of Allergy*, *27*, 312–324.

Harrison, F. C. (1987). Dependency–responsibility–morality: A metapsychological synthesis. *American Journal of Social Psychiatry*, *7*, 245–252.

Hartup, W. W. (1963). Dependence and independence. In H. W. Stevenson (Ed.), *Child psychology* (pp. 333–363). Washington, DC: National Society for the Study of Education.

Hartup, W. W., & Keller, E. D. (1960). Nurturance in preschool children and its relation to dependency. *Child Development*, *31*, 681–689.

Hatfield, J. S., Ferguson, P. E., Rau, L., & Alpert, R. (1967). Mother–child interaction and the socialization process. *Child Development*, *38*, 365–414.

Hayakawa, M. (1977). A study of identity status in the relationship between self-concept and dependency in adolescence. *Tohoku Psychologica Folia*, *36*, 23–31.

Hayward, C., & King, R. (1990). Somatization and personality disorder traits in nonclinical volunteers. *Journal of Personality Disorders, 4,* 402–406.

Hazan, C., & Shaver, P. (1987). Romantic love conceptualized as an attachment process. *Journal of Personality and Social Psychology, 52,* 511–524.

Head, S. B., Baker, J. D., & Williamson, D. A. (1991). Family environment characteristics and dependent personality disorder. *Journal of Personality Disorders, 5,* 256–263.

Heathers, G. (1953). Emotional dependence and independence in a physical threat situation. *Child Development, 24,* 169–179.

Heathers, G. (1955a). Acquiring dependence and independence: A theoretical orientation. *Journal of Genetic Psychology, 87,* 277–291.

Heathers, G. (1955b). Emotional dependence and independence in nursery school play. *Journal of Genetic Psychology, 87,* 37–57.

Hedayat, M. M., & Kelly, D. B. (1991). Relationship of MMPI dependency and dominance scale scores to staff's ratings, diagnoses, and demographic data for day-treatment clients. *Psychological Reports, 68,* 259–266.

Heinstein, M. I. (1963). Behavioral correlates of breast–bottle regimes under varying parent–infant relationships. *Monographs of the Society for Research in Child Development, 28,* 1–61.

Heller, K., & Goldstein, A. P. (1961). Client dependency and therapist expectancy as relationship-maintaining variables in psychotherapy. *Journal of Consulting Psychology, 25,* 371–375.

Helson, R., & Wink, P. (1992). Personality change in women from the early 40s to the early 50s. *Psychology and Aging, 7,* 46–55.

Henderson, S. (1974). Care-eliciting behavior in man. *Journal of Nervous and Mental Disease, 159,* 172–181.

Hendrick, C., & Hendrick, S. S. (1989). Research on love: Does it measure up? *Journal of Personality and Social Psychology, 56,* 784–794.

Hiler, E. W. (1959). The sentence completion test as a predictor of continuation in psychotherapy. *Journal of Consulting Psychology, 23,* 544–549.

Hirschfeld, R. M. A., Klerman, G. L., Andreason, N. C., Clayton, P. J., & Keller, M. B. (1986). Psychosocial predictors of chronicity in depressed patients. *British Journal of Psychiatry, 148,* 648–654.

Hirschfeld, R. M. A., Klerman, G. L., Clayton, P. J., & Keller, M. B. (1983). Personality and depression: Empirical findings. *Archives of General Psychiatry, 40,* 993–998.

Hirschfeld, R. M. A., Klerman, G. L., Clayton, P. J., Keller, M. B., & Andreason, N. C. (1984). Personality and gender-related differences in depression. *Journal of Affective Disorders, 7,* 211–221.

Hirschfeld, R. M. A., Klerman, G. L., Gough, H. G., Barrett, J., Korchin, S. J., & Chodoff, P. (1977). A measure of interpersonal dependency. *Journal of Personality Assessment, 41,* 610–618.

Hirschfeld, R. M. A., Klerman, G. L., Lavori, P., Keller, M. B., Griffith, P., & Coryell, W. (1989). Premorbid personality assessments of first onset of major depression. *Archives of General Psychiatry, 46,* 345–350.

Hirschfeld, R. M. A., Shea, M. T., & Weise, R. (1991). Dependent personality disorder: Perspectives for DSM-IV. *Journal of Personality Disorders, 5,* 135–149.

Hoare, P. (1984). Does illness foster dependency? A study of epileptic and diabetic children. *Developmental Medicine and Child Neurology, 16,* 20–24.

Hoffman, J. A. (1984). Psychological separation of late adolescents from their parents. *Journal of Counseling Psychology, 31,* 170–178.

Hoffman, J. A., & Weiss, B. (1987). Family dynamics and presenting problems in college students. *Journal of Counseling Psychology, 34,* 157–163.

Hokanson, J. E., & Butler, A. C. (1992). Cluster analysis of depressed college students' social behaviors. *Journal of Personality and Social Psychology, 62,* 273–280.

Holden, R. R., & Reddon, J. R. (1987). Temporal personality variations among participants from a university subject pool. *Psychological Reports, 60,* 1247–1254.

Hollender, M. C., Luborsky, L., & Harvey, R. (1970). Correlates of the desire to be held in women. *Journal of Psychosomatic Research, 14,* 387–390.

Holt, R. R. (1966). Measuring libidinal and aggressive motives and their controls by means of the Rorschach test. In D. Levine (Ed.), *Nebraska symposium on motivation* (Vol. 14, pp. 1–47). Lincoln, NE: University of Nebraska Press.

Hopkins, L. B. (1986). Dependency issues and fears in long-term psychotherapy. *Psychotherapy, 23,* 535–539.

Horney, K. (1945). *Our inner conflicts.* New York: W. W. Norton.

Horowitz, I. A. (1968). Effect of choice and locus of dependence on helping behavior. *Journal of Personality and Social Psychology, 8,* 373–376.

Hull, C. L. (1943). *Principles of behavior.* New York: Appleton-Century-Crofts.

Hunt, E., Browning, P., & Nave, G. (1982). A behavioral exploration of dependent and independent mildly mentally retarded adolescents and their mothers. *Applied Research in Mental Retardation, 3,* 141–150.

Hyler, S. E., Rieder, R. O., Williams, J. B. W., Spitzer, R. L., Hendler, J., & Lyons, M. (1988). The Personality Diagnostic Questionnaire. *Journal of Personality Disorders, 2,* 229–237.

Hyler, S. E., Skodol, A. E., Kellman, H. D., Oldham, J. M., & Rosnick, L. (1990). Validity of the Personality Diagnostic Questionnaire—Revised: Comparison with two structured interviews. *American Journal of Psychiatry, 147,* 1043–1048.

Iga, M. (1966). Relation of suicide attempt and social structure in Kamakura, Japan. *International Journal of Social Psychiatry, 12,* 221–232.

Ihilevich, D., & Gleser, G. C. (1986). *Defense mechanisms.* Owosso, MI: DMI Associates.

Jackson, H. J., Gazis, J., Rudd, R. P., & Edwards, J. (1991a). Concordance between two personality disorder instruments with psychiatric inpatients. *Comprehensive Psychiatry, 32,* 252–260.

Jackson, H. J., Rudd, R., Gazis, J., & Edwards, J. (1991b). Using the MCMI to diagnose personality disorders in inpatients: Axis I/Axis II associations and sex differences. *Australian Psychologist, 26,* 37–41.

Jackson, H. J., Whiteside, H. L., Bates, G. W., Bell, R., Rudd, R. P., & Edwards, J. (1991c). Diagnosing personality disorders in psychiatric inpatients. *Acta Psychiatrica Scandinavica, 83,* 206–213.

Jackson, J. M., Procidano, M. E., & Cohen, C. J. (1989). Subject pool sign-up procedures: A threat to external validity. *Social Behavior and Personality*, *17*, 29–43.

Jacobs, M. A., Anderson, L. S., Champagne, E., Karush, N., Richman, S. J., & Knapp, P. H. (1966). Orality, impulsivity and cigarette smoking in men. *Journal of Nervous and Mental Disease*, *143*, 207–219.

Jacobs, M. A., Knapp, P. H., Anderson, L. S., Karush, N., Meissner, R., & Richman, S. J. (1965). Relationship of oral frustration factors with heavy cigarette smoking in males. *Journal of Nervous and Mental Disease*, *141*, 161–171.

Jacobs, M. A., & Spilken, A. Z. (1971). Personality patterns associated with heavy cigarette smoking in male college students. *Journal of Consulting and Clinical Psychology*, *37*, 428–432.

Jacobson, R., & Robins, C. J. (1989). Social dependency and social support in bulimic and nonbulimic women. *International Journal of Eating Disorders*, *8*, 665–670.

Jakubczak, L. F., & Walters, R. H. (1959). Suggestibility as dependency behavior. *Journal of Abnormal and Social Psychology*, *59*, 102–107.

Jamison, K., & Comrey, A. L. (1968). Further study of dependence as a personality factor. *Psychological Reports*, *22*, 239–242.

Jemmot, J. B., & Locke, S. E. (1984). Psychosocial factors, immunological mediation, and human susceptibility to infectious diseases. *Psychological Bulletin*, *95*, 78–108.

Jessor, R., & Jessor, S. L. (1977). *Problem behavior and psychosocial development*. New York: Academic Press.

Joffe, R. T., & Regan, J. J. (1988). Personality and depression. *Journal of Psychiatric Research*, *22*, 279–286.

Joffe, R. T., Swinson, R. P., & Regan, J. J. (1988). Personality features of obsessive–compulsive disorder. *American Journal of Psychiatry*, *145*, 1127–1129.

Jones, E., Wells, H., & Torrey, R. (1958). Some effects of feedback from the experimenter on conformity behavior. *Journal of Abnormal and Social Psychology*, *57*, 207–213.

Jones, E. E., & Pittman, T. S. (1982). Toward a general theory of strategic self-presentation. In J. Suls (Ed.), *Psychological perspectives on the self* (pp. 231–262). Hillsdale, NJ: Erlbaum.

Jones, M. B. (1957). The Pensacola Z survey: A study in the measurement of authoritarian tendency. *Psychological Monographs*, *71*, 1–19.

Jones, M. C. (1968). Personality correlates and antecedents of drinking patterns in adult males. *Journal of Consulting and Clinical Psychology*, *32*, 2–12.

Jones, M. C. (1971). Personality antecedents and correlates of drinking patterns in women. *Journal of Consulting and Clinical Psychology*, *36*, 61–69.

Jones, R. A. (1970). Volunteering to help. *Journal of Personality and Social Psychology*, *14*, 121–129.

Juni, S. (1981). Maintaining anonymity vs requesting feedback as a function of oral dependency. *Perceptual and Motor Skills*, *52*, 239–242.

Juni, S., & Fischer, R. E. (1983). Religiosity and preoedipal fixation. *Journal of Genetic Psychology*, *146*, 27–35.

Juni, S., & LoCascio, R. (1985). Preference for counseling and psychotherapy as related to preoedipal fixation. *Psychological Reports*, *56*, 431–438.

Juni, S., Masling, J. M., & Brannon, R. (1979). Interpersonal touching and orality. *Journal of Personality Assessment, 43,* 235–237.

Juni, S., Nelson, S. P., & Brannon, R. (1986). Minor tonality music preference and oral dependency. *Journal of Psychology, 121,* 229–236.

Juni, S., & Semel, S. R. (1982). Person perception as a function of orality and anality. *Journal of Social Psychology, 118,* 99–103.

Kagan, J., & Freeman, M. (1963). Relation of childhood intelligence, maternal behaviors and social class to behavior during adolescence. *Child Development, 34,* 899–911.

Kagan, J., & Moss, H. A. (1960). The stability of passive and dependent behavior from childhood through adulthood. *Child Development, 31,* 577–591.

Kagan, J., & Moss, H. A. (1962). *From birth to maturity.* New York: Wiley.

Kagan, J., & Mussen, P. (1956). Dependency themes on the TAT and group conformity. *Journal of Consulting Psychology, 20,* 29–32.

Kalish, R. A. (1969). *The dependencies of old people.* Ann Arbor, MI: University of Michigan Institute of Gerontology.

Kalmuss, D. S., & Straus, M. A. (1982). Wife's marital dependency and wife abuse. *Journal of Marriage and the Family, 44,* 277–286.

Kammeier, M. L., Hoffman, H., & Loper, R. G. (1973). Personality characteristics of alcoholics as college freshman and at time of treatment. *Quarterly Journal of Studies on Alcohol, 34,* 390–399.

Kanter, V. B., & Hazelton, J. E. (1964). An attempt to measure some aspects of personality in young men with duodenal ulcer by means of questionnaires and a projective test. *Journal of Psychosomatic Research, 8,* 297–309.

Kaplan, M. (1983). A woman's view of DSM-III. *American Psychologist, 38,* 786–792.

Karasawa, K. (1991). The effects of onset and offest reponsibility on affects and helping judgments. *Journal of Applied Social Psychology, 21,* 482–499.

Kardiner, A. (1939). *The individual and his society.* New York: Columbia University Press.

Kass, F., Spitzer, R. L., & Williams, J. B. W. (1983). An empirical study of the issue of sex bias in the diagnostic criteria of DSM-III Axis II personality disorders. *American Psychologist, 38,* 799–801.

Kaul, V., Mathur, P., & Murlidharan, R. (1982). Dependency and its antecedents: A review. *Indian Educational Review, 17,* 35–46.

Keinan, G., & Hobfoll, S. E. (1989). Stress, dependency and social support: Who benefits from husband's presence in delivery? *Journal of Social and Clinical Psychology, 8,* 32–44.

Keith, R. R., & Vandenberg, S. G. (1974). Relation between orality and weight. *Psychological Reports, 35,* 1205–1206.

Kelley, H. H. (1973). The process of causal attribution. *American Psychologist, 28,* 107–128.

Kelly, J. A., & Worrell, L. (1976). Parental behaviors related to masculine, feminine and androgenous sex role orientations. *Journal of Consulting and Clinical Psychology, 44,* 843–851.

Kernberg, O. (1976). *Object relations theory and clinical psychoanalysis.* New York: Jason Aronson.

Kertzman, D. (1980). *Dependency, frustration tolerance and impulse control in child abusers*. Saratoga, CA: Century Twenty-One.

Khampalikit, S. (1983). The interrelationships between the asthmatic child's dependency behavior, his perception of his illness, and his mother's perception of his illness. *Maternal-Child Nursing Journal, 12*, 221–295.

Khan, S. A., & Sinha, J. B. P. (1971). Social anxiety in dependence-prone persons. *Psychological Studies, 16*, 42–44.

Khantzian, E. J., & Treece, C. (1985). DSM-III psychiatric diagnosis of narcotic addicts: Recent findings. *Archives of General Psychiatry, 42*, 1067–1071.

Kiecolt-Glaser, J. K., Fisher, L., Ogrocki, P., Stout, J. C., Speicher, C. E., & Glaser, R. (1987). Marital quality, marital disruption and immune function. *Psychosomatic Medicine, 49*, 13–34.

Kihlstrom, J. F., & Cantor, N. (1984). Mental representations of the self. In L. Berkowitz (Ed.), *Advances in experimental social psychology* (Vol. 17, pp. 1–47). New York: Academic Press.

Kilbourne, B. K., & Kilbourne, M. T. (1983). Concurrent feelings of power and dependency in a sheltered workshop for chronic neuropsychiatrics. *International Journal of Social Psychiatry, 29*, 173–179.

Kimeldorf, C., & Gewitz, P. J. (1966). Smoking and the Blacky orality factors. *Journal of Projective Techniques, 30*, 167–168.

Klein, D. N. (1989). The Depressive Experiences Questionnaire: A further evaluation. *Journal of Personality Assessment, 53*, 703–715.

Klein, D. N., Harding, K., Taylor, E. B., & Dickstein, S. (1988). Dependency and self-criticism in depression: Evaluation in a clinical population. *Journal of Abnormal Psychology, 97*, 399–404.

Kleiner, L., & Marshall, W. L. (1985). Relationship difficulties and agoraphobia. *Clinical Psychology Review, 5*, 581–595.

Kline, P., & Storey, R. (1977). A factor-analytic study of the oral character. *British Journal of Social and Clinical Psychology, 16*, 317–328.

Kline, P., & Storey, R. (1980). The etiology of the oral character. *Journal of Genetic Psychology, 136*, 85–94.

Kobayashi, J. S. (1989). Depathologizing dependency: Two perspectives. *Psychiatric Annals, 19*, 653–658.

Koenigsberg, H. W., Kaplan, R. D., Gilmore, M. M., & Cooper, A. M. (1985). The relationship between syndrome and personality disorder in DSM-III: Experience with 2,462 patients. *American Journal of Psychiatry, 142*, 207–212.

Kosten, T. R., Rounsaville, B. J., & Kleber, H. D. (1982). DSM-III personality disorders in opiate addicts. *Comprehensive Psychiatry, 23*, 572–581.

Kraeplin, E. (1913). *Psychiatrie: Ein lehrbuch*. Leipzig: Barth.

Krebs, D. R. (1970). Altruism: An examination of the concept and a review of the literature. *Psychological Bulletin, 73*, 258–302.

Lacey, J. H., Coker, S., & Birtchnell, S. A. (1986). Bulimia: Factors associated with its etiology and maintenance. *International Journal of Eating Disorders, 5*, 475–487.

Landrine, H. (1989). The politics of personality disorder. *Psychology of Women Quarterly, 13*, 325–339.

Langveld, J. (1954). The form in which allergic manifestations present themselves to the psychologist during the psychological examination of children. *International Archives of Allergy and Applied Immunology*, 5, 314–315.

Lansky, L. M., Crandall, V. J., Kagan, J., & Baker, C. T. (1961). Sex differences in aggression and its correlates in middle-class adolescents. *Child Development*, 32, 45–58.

Lao, R. C. (1980). Differential factors affecting male and female academic performance in high school. *Journal of Psychology*, 104, 119–127.

Lapan, R., & Patton, M. J. (1986). Self-psychology and the adolescent process: Measures of pseudoautonomy and peer-group dependence. *Journal of Counseling Psychology*, 33, 136–142.

Lauer, J. W. (1976). The effect of tricyclic antidepressant compounds on patients with passive–dependent personality traits. *Current Therapeutic Research*, 19, 495–505.

Laury, G. V. (1970). The battered child syndrome: Parental motivation and clinical aspects. *Bulletin of the New York Academy of Medicine*, 46, 676–684.

Lawlis, G. F., & Rubin, S. E. (1971). A 16PF study of personality patterns in alcoholics. *Quarterly Journal of Studies on Alcohol*, 32, 318–327.

Lazare, A., Klerman, G. L., & Armor, D. J. (1966). Oral, obsessive and hysterical personality patterns. *Archives of General Psychiatry*, 14, 624–630.

Lazare, A., Klerman, G. L., & Armor, D. J. (1970). Oral, obsessive and hysterical personality patterns: Replication of factor analysis in an independent sample. *Journal of Psychiatric Research*, 7, 275–290.

Leary, M. R. (1983). A brief version of the Fear of Negative Evaluation scale. *Personality and Social Psychology Bulletin*, 9, 371–375.

Leary, T. (1957). *Interpersonal diagnosis of personality*. New York: Ronald.

Lemert, E. M. (1962). Dependency in married alcoholics. *Quarterly Journal of Studies on Alcohol*, 23, 590–609.

Lenihan, G. O., & Kirk, W. G. (1990). Personality characteristics of eating-disordered outpatients as measured by the Hand Test. *Journal of Personality Assessment*, 55, 350–361.

Lerner, H. E. (1983). Female dependency in context: Some theoretical and technical considerations. *American Journal of Orthopsychiatry*, 53, 697–705.

LeShan, L. L., & Worthington, R. E. (1956). Loss of cathexes as a common psychodynamic indicator of cancer patients. *Psychological Reports*, 2, 183–193.

Lester, D. (1969). Resentment and dependency in the suicidal individual. *Journal of General Psychology*, 81, 137–145.

Levin, A. P., & Hyler, S. E. (1986). DSM-III personality diagnosis in bulimia. *Comprehensive Psychiatry*, 27, 47–53.

Levine, S., Wiener, S. G., & Coe, C. (1989). The psychoneuroendocrinology of stress. In F. R. Brush & S. Levine (Eds.), *Psychoendocrinology* (pp. 341–377). New York: Academic Press.

Levit, D. B. (1991). Gender differences in ego defenses in adolescence. *Journal of Personality and Social Psychology*, 61, 992–999.

Levitt, E. E., Lubin, B., & Zuckerman, M. A. (1962). A simplified method for scoring Rorschach content for dependency. *Journal of Projective Techniques*, 26, 234–236.

Levy, D. M. (1943). *Maternal overprotection*. New York: Columbia University Press.

Lewin, K. (1951). Problems of research in social psychology. In D. Cartwright (Ed.), *Field theory in social science* (pp. 155–169). New York: Harper & Row.

Libby, W. L., & Yanklevich, D. (1973). Personality determinants of eye contact and direction of gaze aversion. *Journal of Personality and Social Psychology, 27,* 197–206.

Lindzey, G. (1959). On the classification of projective techniques. *Psychological Bulletin, 56,* 156–168.

Linke, S., & Taylor, D. (1987). Levels of dependency of the long-term mentally disabled in community and hospital settings. *Behavioral Psychotherapy, 15,* 314–318.

Livesley, W. J., Jackson, D. J., & Schroeder, M. L. (1989). A study of the factorial structure of personality pathology. *Journal of Personality Disorders, 3,* 292–306.

Livesley, W. J., Schroeder, M. L., & Jackson, D. N. (1990). Dependent personality disorder and attachment problems. *Journal of Personality Disorders, 4,* 131–140.

Lomas, P. (1965). Passivity and failure of identity development. *International Journal of Psycho-Analysis, 46,* 438–454.

Loring, M., & Powell, B. (1988). Gender, race and DSM-III: A study of the objectivity of psychiatric diagnostic behavior. *Journal of Health and Social Behavior, 29,* 1–22.

Lorr, M., & McNair, D. M. (1964a). Correlates of length of psychotherapy. *Journal of Clinical Psychology, 20,* 497–504.

Lorr, M., & McNair, D. M. (1964b). The interview relationship in therapy. *Journal of Nervous and Mental Disease, 139,* 328–331.

Lorr, M., Youniss, R. P., & Kluth, C. (1992). The Interpersonal Style Inventory and the five-factor model. *Journal of Clinical Psychology, 48,* 202–206.

Lower, R. (1967). Psychotherapy of neurotic dependency. *American Journal of Psychiatry, 124,* 100–104.

Lubin, B., Larsen, R. M., & Matarazzo, J. D. (1984). Patterns of psychological test usage in the United States, 1935–1982. *American Psychologist, 39,* 451–454.

Luborsky, L., & Auerbach, A. H. (1969). The symptom–context method. *Journal of the American Psychoanalytic Association, 17,* 68–99.

Lyon, D., & Greenberg, J. (1991). Evidence of co-dependency in women with an alcoholic parent. *Journal of Personality and Social Psychology, 61,* 435–439.

Lytton, H., & Romney, D. M. (1991). Parents' differential socialization of boys and girls: A meta-analysis. *Psychological Bulletin, 109,* 267–296.

Maccoby, E. E. (1980). *Social development*. New York: Harcourt-Brace.

Maccoby, E. E., & Jacklin, C. N. (1974). *The psychology of sex differences*. Stanford, CA: Stanford University Press.

Maccoby, E. E., & Masters, J. C. (1970). Attachment and dependency. In P. H. Mussen (Ed.), *Carmichael's manual of child psychology* (Vol 2, pp. 73–157). New York: Wiley.

Magni, G., DiMario, F., Rizzardo, R., Pulin, S., & Naccarato, R. (1986). Personality profiles of patients with duodenal ulcer. *American Journal of Psychiatry, 143,* 1297–1300.

Magni, G., Rizzardo, R., & DiMario, F. (1984). Personality and psychological factors in chronic duodenal ulcer. *Archives of Neurology and Psychiatry, 135,* 315–320.

Magni, G., Salmi, A., & Paterlini, A. (1982). Psychological distress in duodenal ulcer and acute gastroduodenitis. *Digestive Science, 27,* 1081–1084.

Mahler, M. S., Pine, F., & Bergman, A. (1975). *The psychological birth of the human infant.* New York: Basic Books.

Mahon, N. E. (1982). The relationship of self-disclosure, interpersonal dependency and life changes to loneliness in young adults. *Nursing Research, 31,* 343–347.

Main, M., Kaplan, N., & Cassidy, J. (1985). Security in infancy, childhood and adulthood. *Monographs of the Society for Research in Child Development, 50,* 66–104.

Mann, R. D. (1959). A review of the relationships between personality and performance in small groups. *Psychological Bulletin, 56,* 241–270.

Marcus, R. F. (1975). The child as elicitor of parental sanctions for independent and dependent behavior. *Developmental Psychology, 11,* 443–452.

Marcus, R. F. (1976). The effects of children's emotional and instrumental dependent behavior on parental response. *Journal of Psychology, 92,* 57–63.

Marsh, D. T., Stile, S. A., Stoughton, N. L., & Trout-Landen, B. L. (1988). Psychopathology of opiate addiction: Comparative data from the MMPI and MCMI. *American Journal of Drug and Alcohol Abuse, 14,* 17–27.

Marshall, H. R., & McCandless, B. R. (1957). Relationships between dependence on adults and social acceptance by peers. *Child Development, 28,* 413–419.

Marshall, J. R., & Neill, J. (1977). The removal of a psychosomatic symptom: Effects on the marriage. *Family Process, 16,* 273–280.

Masling, J. M. (1986). Orality, pathology and interpersonal behavior. In J. Masling (Ed.), *Empirical studies of psychoanalytic theories* (Vol. 2, pp. 73–106). Hillsdale, NJ: Erlbaum.

Masling, J. M., Bornstein, R. F., Poynton, F. G., Reed, S. D., & Katkin, E. S. (1991). Perception without awareness and electrodermal responding. *Journal of Mind and Behavior, 12,* 33–48.

Masling, J. M., Johnson, C., & Saturansky, C. (1974). Oral imagery, accuracy of perceiving others and performance in Peace Corps training. *Journal of Personality and Social Psychology, 30,* 414–419.

Masling, J. M., O'Neill, R. M., & Jayne, C. (1981). Orality and latency of volunteering to serve as experimental subjects. *Journal of Personality Assessment, 45,* 20–22.

Masling, J. M., O'Neill, R. M., & Katkin, E. S. (1982). Autonomic arousal, interpersonal climate and orality. *Journal of Personality and Social Psychology, 42,* 529–534.

Masling, J. M., Price, J., Goldband, S., & Katkin, E. S. (1981). Oral imagery and autonomic arousal in social isolation. *Journal of Personality and Social Psychology, 40,* 395–400.

Masling, J. M., Rabie, L., & Blondheim, S. H. (1967). Obesity, level of aspiration, and Rorschach and TAT measures of oral dependence. *Journal of Consulting Psychology, 31,* 233–239.

Masling, J. M., Schiffner, J., & Shenfeld, M. (1980). Client perception of the therapist, orality, and sex of client and therapist. *Journal of Counseling Psychology*, *27*, 294–298.

Masling, J. M., & Schwartz, M. A. (1979). A critique of research in psychoanalytic theory. *Genetic Psychology Monographs*, *100*, 257–307.

Masling, J. M., Weiss, L., & Rothschild, B. (1968). Relationships of oral imagery to yielding behavior and birth order. *Journal of Consulting and Clinical Psychology*, *32*, 89–91.

Maslow, A. H. (1970). *Motivation and personality*. New York: Harper.

Mathes, E. W., Roter, P. M., & Joerger, S. M. (1982). A convergent validity study of six jealousy scales. *Psychological Reports*, *50*, 1143–1147.

Mavissakalian, M., & Hamann, M. S. (1986). DSM-III personality disorder in agoraphobia. *Comprehensive Psychiatry*, *27*, 471–479.

Mavissakalian, M., & Hamann, M. S. (1987). DSM-III personality disorder in agoraphobia, II: Changes with treatment. *Comprehensive Psychiatry*, *28*, 356–361.

May, R. (1969). *Existential psychology*. New York: Random House.

McCandless, B. R., Bilous, C. B., & Bennett, H. L. (1961). Peer popularity and dependence on adults in pre-school-age socialization. *Child Development*, *32*, 511–518.

McCann, J. T. (1991). Convergent and discriminant validity of the MCMI-II and MMPI personality disorder scales. *Psychological Assessment*, *3*, 9–18.

McClain, E. (1978). Feminists and nonfeminists: Contrasting profiles in independence and affiliation. *Psychological Reports*, *43*, 435–441.

McCord, J., McCord, W., & Thurber, E. (1962). Some effects of paternal absence on male children. *Journal of Abnormal and Social Psychology*, *64*, 361–369.

McCranie, E. W., & Bass, J. D. (1984). Childhood family antecedents of dependency and self-criticism. *Journal of Abnormal Psychology*, *93*, 3–8.

McCully, R., Glucksman, M., & Hirsch, J. (1968). Nutrition imagery in the Rorschach materials of food-deprived, obese patients. *Journal of Projective Techniques and Personality Assessment*, *32*, 375–382.

McIntosh, J. H., Nasiry, R. W., & Frysman, M. (1983). The personality pattern of patients with chronic peptic ulcer. *Scandinavian Journal of Gastroenterology*, *18*, 945–950.

McMahon, R. C., Davidson, R. S., Gersh, D., & Flynn, P. (1991). A comparison of continuous and episodic drinkers using the MCMI, MMPI, and ALCE-VAL-R. *Journal of Clinical Psychology*, *47*, 148–159.

McMahon, R. C., Flynn, P. J., & Davidson, R. S. (1985). Stability of the personality and symptom scales of the MCMI. *Journal of Personality Assessment*, *49*, 231–234.

McPartland, J. M., & Epstein, J. L. (1975). *An investigation of the interaction of family and social factors in open school*. Baltimore, MD: Centre for the Social Organization of Schools, Johns Hopkins University.

Meijer, A. (1981). A controlled study of asthmatic children and their families. *Israeli Journal of Psychiatry*, *18*, 197–208.

Mellsop, G., Varghese, F., Joshua, S., & Hicks, A. (1982). The reliability of DSM-III Axis II. *American Journal of Psychiatry*, *139*, 1360–1361.

Melnick, B., & Hurley, J. R. (1969). Distinctive personality attributes of child-abusing mothers. *Journal of Consulting and Clinical Psychology, 33,* 746–749.

Mersky, H., & Trimble, M. (1979). Personality, sexual adjustment, and brain lesions in patients with conversion symptoms. *American Journal of Psychiatry, 136,* 179–182.

Mezzich, J. E., Fabrega, H., & Coffman, G. A. (1987). Multiaxial characteristics of depressive patients. *Journal of Nervous and Mental Disease, 175,* 339–346.

Midlarsky, E. (1971). Aiding under stress: The effects of competence, dependency, visibility and fatalism. *Journal of Personality, 39,* 132–149.

Midlarsky, E., & Midlarsky, M. (1973). Some determinants of aiding under experimentally induced stress. *Journal of Personality, 41,* 305–327.

Miller, D. R., & Stine, M. W. (1951). The prediction of social acceptance by means of psychoanalytic concepts. *Journal of Personality, 20,* 162–174.

Millon, T. (1981). *Disorders of personality: DSM-III Axis 2.* New York: Wiley.

Millon, T. (1987). *Millon Clinical Multiaxial Inventory—II manual.* Minneapolis, MN: National Computer Systems.

Mills, J. K., & Cunningham, J. (1988). Oral character and attitudes and behavior related to food and eating. *Psychological Reports, 63,* 15–18.

Mischel, W. (1970). Sex-typing and socialization. In P. H. Mussen (Ed.), *Carmichael's manual of child psychology* (3rd ed.) (pp. 3–72). New York: Wiley.

Mischel, W. (1973). Toward a cognitive social learning reconceptualization of personality. *Psychological Review, 80,* 252–283.

Mischel, W. (1979). On the interface of cognition and personality: Beyond the person–situation debate. *American Psychologist, 34,* 740–754.

Mischel, W. (1984). Convergences and challenges in the search for consistency. *American Psychologist, 39,* 351–364.

Mischel, W., & Peake, P. K. (1982). Beyond deja vu in the search for cross-situational consistency. *Psychological Review, 89,* 730–755.

Mongrain, M., & Zuroff, D. C. (1989). Cognitive vulnerability to depressed affect in dependent and self-critical college women. *Journal of Personality Disorders, 3,* 240–251.

Moore, S. G., & Updegraff, R. (1964). Sociometric status of preschool children as related to age, sex, nurturance-giving and dependence. *Child Development, 35,* 519–524.

Moran, J. J., & Carter, D. E. (1991). Comparisons among children's responses to the Hand Test by grade, race, sex and social class. *Journal of Clinical Psychology, 47,* 647–664.

Moran, L. J., Fairweather, G. W., Fisher, S., & Morton, R. B. (1956). Psychological concomitants to recovery from tuberculosis. *Journal of Consulting Psychology, 20,* 199–203.

Morey, L. C. (1988). A psychometric analysis of the DSM-III-R personality disorder criteria. *Journal of Personality Disorders, 2,* 109–124.

Morey, L. C., Waugh, M. W., & Blashfield, R. K. (1985). MMPI scales for DSM-III personality disorders: Their derivation and correlates. *Journal of Personality Assessment, 49,* 245–251.

Morgan, J. P. (1991). What is co-dependency? *Journal of Clinical Psychology, 47,* 720–729.

Morrison, J. K., Bushell, J. D., Hanson, G. D., Fentiman, J. R., & Holdridge-Crane, S. (1977). Relationship between psychiatric patients' attitudes toward mental illness and attitudes of dependence. *Psychological Reports, 41*, 1194.

Mosbach, P., & Leventhal, H. (1988). Peer group identification and smoking: Implications for intervention. *Journal of Abnormal Psychology, 97*, 238–245.

Moskowitz, D. S. (1982). Coherence and cross-situational generality in personality: A new analysis of old problems. *Journal of Personality and Social Psychology, 43*, 754–768.

Mowrer, O. H. (1950). *Learning theory and personality dynamics*. New York: Ronald.

Murphy, L. B. (1962). *The widening world of childhood*. New York: Basic Books.

Murray, H. A. (1938). *Explorations in personality*. New York: Oxford University Press.

Mussen, P. (1961). Some antecedents and consequences of masculine sex-typing in adolescent boys. *Psychological Monographs, 75* (2, Whole No. 506).

Nace, E. P., Davis, C. W., & Gaspari, J. P. (1991). Axis II comorbidity in substance abusers. *American Journal of Psychiatry, 148*, 118–120.

Nacev, V. (1980). Dependency and ego strength as indicators of patients' attendance in psychotherapy. *Journal of Clinical Psychology, 36*, 691–695.

Nakao, K., Gunderson, J. G., Phillips, K. A., Tanaka, N., Kazuhiro, Y., Takaishi, J., & Nishimura, T. (1992). Functional impairment in personality disorders. *Journal of Personality Disorders, 6*, 24–33.

Navran, L. (1954). A rationally derived MMPI scale to measure dependence. *Journal of Consulting Psychology, 18*, 192.

Neki, J. S. (1976a). An examination of the cultural relativism of dependence as a dynamic of social and therapeutic relationships, I: Socio-developmental. *British Journal of Medical Psychology, 49*, 1–10.

Neki, J. S. (1976b). An examination of the cultural relativism of dependence as a dynamic of social and therapeutic relationships, II: Therapeutic. *British Journal of Medical Psychology, 49*, 11–22.

Nietzel, M. T., & Harris, M. J. (1990). Relationship of dependency and achievement/autonomy to depression. *Clinical Psychology Review, 10*, 279–297.

Noblin, C., Timmons, E., & Kael, H. (1966). Differential effects of positive and negative verbal reinforcement on psychoanalytic character types. *Journal of Personality and Social Psychology, 4*, 224–228.

Novy, D. M. (1992). Psychometric properties of the Interpersonal Style Inventory. *Journal of Clinical Psychology, 48*, 308–314.

Nurnberg, H. G., Raskin, M., Levine, P. E., Pollack, S., Siegel, O., & Prince, R. (1991). The comorbidity of borderline personality disorder and other DSM-III-R Axis II personality disorders. *American Journal of Psychiatry, 148*, 1371–1377.

O'Brien, P. E., & Gaborit, M. (1992). Codependency: A disorder separate from chemical dependency. *Journal of Clinical Psychology, 48*, 129–136.

O'Gorman, P. (1991). Codependency in women. In N. Vandenbergh (Ed.), *Feminist perspectives on addictions* (pp. 153–166). New York: Springer-Verlag.

Ojha, H. (1972). The relation of prestige suggestion to rigidity and dependence proneness. *Journal of Psychological Research, 16*, 70–73.

Ojha, H., & Singh, R. I. P. (1972). Personality factors and marriage role attitudes. *Psychological Studies, 17,* 13–16.

Ojha, H., & Singh, R. R. (1985). Relationship of marriage role attitude with dependence proneness and insecurity in university students. *Psychologia, 28,* 249–253.

Ojha, H., & Singh, R. R. (1988). Childrearing attitudes as related to insecurity and dependence proneness. *Psychological Studies, 33,* 75–79.

Ojha, R. S. (1978). Reaction time as a function of dependence proneness. *Journal of Psychological Research, 22,* 151–152.

Oldham, J. M., Skodol, A. E., Kellman, H. D., Hyler, S. E., Rosnick, L., & Davies, M. (1992). Diagnosis of DSM-III-R personality disorders by two structured interviews: Patterns of comorbidity. *American Journal of Psychiatry, 149,* 213–220.

O'Leary, A. (1990). Stress, emotion and human immune function. *Psychological Bulletin, 108,* 363–382.

O'Neill, R. M., & Bornstein, R. F. (1990). Oral dependence and gender: Factors in help-seeking response set and self-reported psychopathology in psychiatric inpatients. *Journal of Personality Assessment, 55,* 28–40.

O'Neill, R. M., & Bornstein, R. F. (1991). Orality and depression in psychiatric inpatients. *Journal of Personality Disorders, 5,* 1–7.

O'Neill, R. M., Greenberg, R. P., & Fisher, S. (1984). Orality and field dependence. *Psychoanalytic Psychology, 1,* 335–344.

Osofsky, J. D., & O'Connell, E. J. (1972). Parent–child interaction: Daughters' effects upon mothers' and fathers' behaviors. *Developmental Psychology, 7,* 157–168.

Overholser, J. C. (1987). Facilitating autonomy in passive–dependent persons: An integrative model. *Journal of Contemporary Psychotherapy, 17,* 250–269.

Overholser, J. C. (1990). Retest reliabilty of the Millon Clinical Multiaxial Inventory. *Journal of Personality Assessment, 55,* 202–208.

Overholser, J. C. (1991). Categorical assessment of dependent personality disorder in depressed inpatients. *Journal of Personality Disorders, 5,* 243–255.

Overholser, J. C. (1992). Interpersonal dependency and social loss. *Personality and Individual Differences, 13,* 17–23.

Overholser, J. C., Kabakoff, R., & Norman, W. H. (1989). The assessment of personality characteristics in depressed and dependent psychiatric inpatients. *Journal of Personality Assessment, 53,* 40–50.

Paffanbarger, R. S., Wolf, P. A., Notkin, J., & Thorne, M. C. (1966). Chronic disease in former college students: Early predictors of fatal coronary heart disease. *American Journal of Epidemiology, 83,* 314–319.

Pakes, E. H. (1975). Dependency and psychotherapy: Developmental considerations. *American Journal of Psychotherapy, 29,* 128–133.

Pallis, D. J., & Birtchnell, J. (1976). Personality and suicidal history in psychiatric patients. *Journal of Clinical Psychology, 32,* 246–253.

Pandey, J. (1977). Effects of leadership role-playing on dependence proneness responses. *Journal of Social and Educational Studies, 5,* 111–116.

Pandey, J., & Griffitt, W. (1977). Benefactor's sex and nurturance need, recipient's dependency, and the effect of number of potential helpers on helping behavior. *Journal of Personality, 45,* 79–99.

Pareek, U., & Rao, T. V. (1971). *A study of teacher behavior and student mental health.* New Delhi: National Institute of Health.

Parens, H., & Saul, L. J. (1971). *Dependence in man.* New York: International Universities Press.

Parker, G. (1979a). Parental characteristics in relation to depressive disorders. *British Journal of Psychiatry, 134,* 138–147.

Parker, G. (1979b). Reported parental characteristics in relation to trait depression and anxiety levels in a non-clinical group. *Australian and New Zealand Journal of Psychiatry, 13,* 260–264.

Parker, G. (1981). Parental reports of depressives. *Journal of Affective Disorders, 3,* 131–140.

Parker, G. (1983). *Parental overprotection.* New York: Grune and Stratton.

Parker, G., & Lipscombe, P. (1980). The relevance of early parental experiences to adult dependency, hypochondriasis and utilization of primary physicians. *British Journal of Medical Psychology, 53,* 355–363.

Parker, G., Tupling, H., & Brown, L. B. (1979). A parental bonding instrument. *British Journal of Medical Psychology, 52,* 1–10.

Parker, S. (1960). The witiko psychosis in the context of Ojibwa personality and culture. *American Anthropologist, 62,* 603–623.

Pendleton, L., Tisdale, M., & Marler, M. (1991). Personality pathology in bulimics versus controls. *Comprehensive Psychiatry, 32,* 516–520.

Pennebaker, J. W., & Beall, S. (1986). Confronting a traumatic event: Toward an understanding of inhibition and disease. *Journal of Abnormal Psychology, 95,* 274–281.

Pennebaker, J. W., Kiecolt-Glaser, J. K., & Glaser, R. (1988). Disclosure of traumas and immune function. *Journal of Consulting and Clinical Psychology, 56,* 239–245.

Pfohl, B., Corgell, W., Zimmerman, M., & Stangl, D. (1986). DSM-III personality disorders: Diagnostic overlap and internal consistency of individual DSM-III criteria. *Comprehensive Psychiatry, 27,* 21–34.

Phillips, D. L. (1965). Self-reliance and the inclination to adopt the sick role. *Social Forces, 43,* 555–563.

Piersma, H. L. (1987). The MCMI as a measure of DSM-III Axis II diagnoses: An empirical comparison. *Journal of Clinical Psychology, 43,* 478–483.

Pillemer, K. (1985). The dangers of dependency: New findings on domestic violence against the elderly. *Social Problems, 33,* 146–158.

Pilkonis, P. A. (1988). Personality prototypes among depressives: Themes of dependency and autonomy. *Journal of Personality Disorders, 2,* 144–152.

Pilkonis, P. A., & Frank, E. (1988). Personality pathology in recurrent depression. *American Journal of Psychiatry, 145,* 435–441.

Pilowski, I. (1979). Personality and depressive illness. *Acta Psychiatrica Scandinavica, 60,* 170–176.

Pilowski, I., & Katsikitis, M. (1983). Depressive illness and dependency. *Acta Psychiatrica Scandinavica, 68,* 11–14.

Pincus, A. L., & Wiggins, J. S. (1990). Interpersonal problems and conceptions of personality disorders. *Journal of Personality Disorders, 4*, 342–352.

Pleck, J. H. (1981). Men's power with women, other men and society. In R. A. Lewis (Ed.), *Men in difficult times: Masculinity today and tomorrow* (pp. 234–244). New York: Prentice-Hall.

Poldrugo, F., & Forti, B. (1988). Personality disorders and alcoholism treatment outcome. *Drug and Alcohol Dependence, 21*, 171–176.

Pollie, D. M. (1964). A projective study of conflict and defense in peptic ulcers and bronchial asthma. *Journal of Projective Techniques and Personality Assessment, 28*, 67–77.

Pomazal, R. J., & Clore, G. L. (1973). Helping on the highway: Effects of dependency and sex. *Journal of Applied Social Psychology, 3*, 150–164.

Ponzetti, J. J., Cate, R. M., & Koval, J. E. (1983). Violence between couples: Profiling the male abuser. *Personnel and Guidance Journal, 61*, 222–224.

Pruitt, W. A., & Vandecastle, R. L. (1962). Dependency measures and welfare chronicity. *Journal of Consulting Psychology, 26*, 559–560.

Pyle, R. L., Mitchell, J. E., & Eckert, E. D. (1981). Bulimia: A report of 34 cases. *Journal of Clinical Psychiatry, 42*, 60–64.

Rado, S. (1928). The problem of melancholia. *International Journal of Psychoanalysis, 9*, 420–436.

Rathbone-McCuan, E., Dyer, L., & Wartman, J. (1991). Double jeopardy: Chemical dependence and codependence in older women. In N. Vandenbergh (Ed.), *Feminist perspectives on addiction* (pp. 101–113). New York: Springer-Verlag.

Reich, J. (1987a). Instruments measuring DSM-III and DSM-III-R personality disorders. *Journal of Personality Disorders, 1*, 220–240.

Reich, J. (1987b). Sex distribution of DSM-III personality disorders in psychiatric outpatients. *American Journal of Psychiatry, 144*, 485–488.

Reich, J. (1987c). Prevalence of DSM-III-R self-defeating (masochistic) personality disorder in normal and outpatient populations. *Journal of Nervous and Mental Disease, 175*, 52–54.

Reich, J., Noyes, R., Hirschfeld, R., Coryell, W., & O'Gorman, T. (1987). State and personality in depressed and panic patients. *American Journal of Psychiatry, 144*, 181–187.

Reich, J., Noyes, R., & Troughton, E. (1987). Dependent personality disorder associated with phobic avoidance in patients with panic disorder. *American Journal of Psychiatry, 144*, 323–326.

Reich, J., & Troughton, E. (1988). Comparison of DSM-III personality disorders in recovered depressed and panic disorder patients. *Journal of Nervous and Mental Disease, 176*, 300–304.

Retzlaff, P. D., & Bromley, S. (1991). A multi-test alcoholic taxonomy: Canonical coefficient clusters. *Journal of Clinical Psychology, 47*, 299–309.

Reusch, J. (1948). The infantile personality: The core problem of psychosomatic medicine. *Psychosomatic Medicine, 10*, 134–144.

Reznikoff, M. (1955). Psychological factors in breast cancer. *Psychosomatic Medicine, 17*, 96.

Rice, K. G. (1992). Separation–individuation and adjustment to college: A longitudinal study. *Journal of Counseling Psychology, 39*, 203–213.

Richman, J. A., & Flaherty, J. A. (1987). Adult psychosocial assets and depressed mood over time: Effects of internalized childhood attachments. *Journal of Nervous and Mental Disease, 175*, 703–712.

Rienzi, B. M., & Scrams, D. J. (1991). Gender stereotypes for paranoid, antisocial, compulsive, dependent and histrionic personality disorders. *Psychological Reports, 69*, 976–978.

Rim, Y. (1981). The use of means of influence according to ordinal position and length of marriage. *Personality and Individual Differences, 2*, 125–127.

Robins, C. J. (1990). Congruence of personality and life events in depression. *Journal of Abnormal Psychology, 99*, 393–397.

Robins, C. J., & Block, P. (1988). Personal vulnerability, life events and depressive symptoms. *Journal of Personality and Social Psychology, 54*, 847–852.

Robins, C. J., Block, P., & Peselow, E. D. (1989). Relations of sociotropic and autonomous personality characteristics to specific symptoms in depressed patients. *Journal of Abnormal Psychology, 98*, 86–87.

Robins, L. N., Helzer, J. E., Weissman, M. M., Orvaschel, H., Gruenberg, E., Burke, J. D., & Regier, D. A. (1984). Lifetime prevalence of specific psychiatric disorders in three sites. *Archives of General Psychiatry, 41*, 949–958.

Roe, A., & Siegelman, M. (1963). Parent–child relation questionnaire. *Child Development, 34*, 355–369.

Rogers, C. R. (1942). *Counseling and psychotherapy.* Boston: Houghton-Mifflin.

Rogers, C. R. (1980). *A way of being.* Boston: Houghton-Mifflin.

Rosenthal, M. K. (1967). The generalization of dependency behavior from mother to stranger. *Journal of Child Psychology and Psychiatry, 8*, 117–133.

Rosenthal, R. (1984). *Meta-analytic procedures for social research.* Beverly Hills, CA: Sage.

Rosenthal, R., & Rosnow, R. L. (1975). *The volunteer subject.* New York: Wiley.

Ross, L. D. (1977). The intuitive psychologist and his shortcomings. In L. Berkowitz (Ed.), *Advances in experimental social psychology* (Vol. 10, pp. 173–220). New York: Academic Press.

Rossman, P. (1984). Assessing different aspects of psychosocial dependency: A new scale and some empirical results. *Studia Psychologica, 26*, 317–322.

Rossman, P. (1988). Interpersonal dependency: A risk factor for depressive disorders? *Psychologische Beitrage, 30*, 18–28.

Rothbart, M. K. (1981). Measurement of temperament in infancy. *Child Development, 52*, 569–578.

Rothstein, C., & Cohen, I. (1958). Hostility and dependency conflicts in peptic ulcer patients. *Psychological Reports, 4*, 555–558.

Rottschafer, R. H., & Renzaglia, G. A. (1962). The relationship of dependent-like verbal behaviors to counselor style and induced set. *Journal of Consulting Psychology, 26*, 172–177.

Rounsaville, B. J., Rosenberger, P., Wilber, C., Weissman, M. M., & Kleber, H. D. (1980). A comparison of the SADS/RDC and the DSM-III: Diagnosing drug abusers. *Journal of Nervous and Mental Disease, 168*, 90–97.

Rounsaville, B. J., Weissman, M. M., Kleber, H., & Wilber, C. (1982). Heterogeneity of psychiatric diagnosis in treated opiate addicts. *Archives of General Psychiatry, 39*, 161–166.

Ruddick, B. (1961). Agoraphobia. *International Journal of Psycho-Analysis, 42*, 537–543.

Ryder, R. D., & Parry-Jones, W. L. (1982). Fear of dependence and its value in working with adolescents. *Journal of Adolescence, 5*, 71–78.

Saha, S., & Sinha, J. B. P. (1973). The transfer of model effects on dependence proneness. *Indian Journal of Psychology, 48*, 23–29.

Salokangas, R. K. R., Rakkolainen, V., & Lehtinen, P. (1980). The psychiatric treatment system as an adaptational treatment structure: A study of dependency in the treatment behavior of schizophrenic patients. *Psychiatrica Fennica, 7*, 99–109.

Sandler, J., & Dare, C. (1970). The psychoanalytic concept of orality. *Journal of Psychosomatic Research, 14*, 211–222.

Sansanwal, D. N., Jarial, G. S., & Dandel, R. (1982). An experimental study of the effect of dependency and adjustment on the achievement of students studying through programmed learning material using different response modes. *Indian Educational Review, 17*, 140–146.

Saviola, M. E. (1981). Personal reflections on physically disabled women and dependency. *Professional Psychology, 12*, 112–117.

Schachter, S. (1959). *The psychology of affiliation*. Stanford, CA: Stanford University Press.

Schafer, R. (1968). *Aspects of internalization*. New York: International Universities Press.

Schaps, E. (1972). Cost, dependency and helping. *Journal of Personality and Social Psychology, 21*, 74–78.

Schlenker, B. R., & Weigold, M. F. (1990). Self-consciousness and self-presentation: Being autonomous versus appearing autonomous. *Journal of Personality and Social Psychology, 59*, 820–828.

Schmale, A. H. (1958). Relationship of separation and depression to disease. *Psychosomatic Medicine, 20*, 259–270.

Schneider, K. (1923). *Die psychopathischen personlichkeiten*. Vienna: Deuticke.

Schopler, J. (1967). An investigation of sex differences on the influence of dependence. *Sociometry, 30*, 50–63.

Schopler, J., & Bateson, N. (1965). The power of dependence. *Journal of Personality and Social Psychology, 2*, 247–254.

Schopler, J., & Matthews, M. W. (1964). The influence of the perceived causal locus of partner's dependence on the use of interpersonal power. *Journal of Personality and Social Psychology, 2*, 609–612.

Sciuto, G., Diaferia, G., Battaglia, M., Perna, G., Gabriele, A., & Bellodi, L. (1991). DSM-III-R personality disorders in panic and obsessive–compulsive disorder: A comparison study. *Comprehensive Psychiatry, 32*, 450–457.

Sears, R. R. (1963). Dependency motivation. In M. R. Jones (Ed.), *Nebraska symposium on motivation* (Vol. 11, pp. 25–64). Lincoln, NE: University of Nebraska Press.

Sears, R. R. (1972). Attachment, dependency and frustration. In J. L. Gewirtz (Ed.), *Attachment and dependency* (pp. 1–27). New York: Wiley.

Sears, R. R., Maccoby, E. E., & Levin, H. (1957). *Patterns of child rearing*. Evanston, IL: Row-Peterson.

Sears, R. R., Rau, L., & Alpert, R. (1965). *Identification and child rearing*. Stanford, CA: Stanford University Press.

Sears, R. R., Whiting, J. W. M., Nowlis, V., & Sears, P. S. (1953). Some childrearing antecedents of aggression and dependency in young children. *Genetic Psychology Monographs, 47*, 135–236.

Sears, R. R., & Wise, G. W. (1950). Relation of cup feeding in infancy to thumbsucking and the oral drive. *American Journal of Orthopsychiatry, 20*, 123–138.

Selvey, C. L. (1973). Concerns about death in relation to sex, dependency, guilt about hostility and feelings of powerlessness. *Omega, 4*, 209–219.

Shafar, S. (1970). Aspects of phobic illness. *British Journal of Medical Psychology, 49*, 211–236.

Sharma, S., & Rao, C. (1974). Personality factors and adjustment patterns of peptic ulcer patients in India. *Psychosomatics, 15*, 139–142.

Shilkret, C. J., & Masling, J. M. (1981). Oral dependence and dependent behavior. *Journal of Personality Assessment, 45*, 125–129.

Siegel, R. J. (1988). Women's dependency in a male-centered value system. *Women and Therapy, 7*, 113–123.

Siegelman, M. (1966). Loving and punishing parental behavior and introversion tendencies in sons. *Child Development, 37*, 985–992.

Silverman, L. H., Lachmann, F. M., & Milich, R. H. (1982). *The search for oneness*. New York: International Universities Press.

Simpson, J. A. (1990). Influence of attachment styles on romantic relationships. *Journal of Personality and Social Psychology, 59*, 971–980.

Simpson, J. A., & Gangestad, S. W. (1991). Individual differences in sociosexuality: Evidence for convergent and discriminant validity. *Journal of Personality and Social Psychology, 60*, 870–883.

Singh, R. R., & Ojha, S. K. (1987). Sex difference in dependence proneness, insecurity and self-concept. *Manas, 34*, 61–66.

Singh, S. (1981). Fear of failure among females as related to personality, locus of control, behavior problems and childrearing practices. *Personality Study and Group Behavior, 1*, 96–108.

Singh, S., & Lunyal, K. (1981). Psychometric and behavioral correlates of a hostile press measure of fear of failure. *Indian Journal of Clinical Psychology, 8*, 101–107.

Sinha, J. B. P. (1968). A test of dependence proneness. *Journal of Psychological Research, 12*, 66–70.

Sinha, J. B. P., & Pandey, J. (1972). The processes of decision making in dependence prone persons. *Journal of Psychological Research, 16*, 35–37.

Smith, A. B., & Bain, H. (1978). Dependency in day-care and playcenter children. *New Zealand Journal of Educational Studies, 13*, 163–173.

Smith, H. T. (1958). A comparison of interview and observation measures of mother behavior. *Journal of Abnormal and Social Psychology, 57*, 278–282.

Smith, T. W., O'Keeffe, J. L., & Jenkins, M. (1988). Dependency and self-criticism: Correlates of depression or moderators of the effects of stressful events? *Journal of Personality Disorders, 2*, 160–169.

Snyder, M. (1981). On the self-perpetuating nature of social stereotypes. In D. L. Hamilton (Ed.), *Cognitive processes in stereotyping and intergroup behavior* (pp. 183–212). Hillsdale, NJ: Erlbaum.

Snyder, W. U. (1963). *Dependency in psychotherapy*. New York: MacMillan.

Spence, D. P. (1970). Human and computer attempts to decode symptom language. *Psychosomatic Medicine, 32*, 615–625.

Spence, J. T., & Helmreich, R. L. (1978). *Masculinity and femininity: Their psychological dimensions, correlates and antecedents*. Austin, TX: University of Texas Press.

Sperling, M. B., & Berman, W. H. (1991). An attachment classification of desparate love. *Journal of Personality Assessment, 56*, 45–55.

Spiesman, J. C., & Singer, M. T. (1961). Rorschach content correlates in five groups with organic pathology. *Journal of Projective Techniques, 25*, 356–359.

Spitz, R. (1965). *The first year of life*. New York: International Universities Press.

Spitzer, R. L., Forman, J. B. W., & Nee, J. (1979). DSM-III field trials, I: Initial interrater diagnostic reliability. *American Journal of Psychiatry, 136*, 815–817.

Spolter, B. M., Tokar, J. T., & Gocka, E. F. (1978). Dependency and alcoholic recidivism. *Psychological Reports, 43*, 538.

Sprock, J., Blashfield, R. K., & Smith, B. (1990). Gender weighting of DSM-III-R personality disorder criteria. *American Journal of Psychiatry, 147*, 586–590.

Sroufe, L. A. (1983). Infant–caregiver attachment and patterns of attachment in preschool. In M. Perlmutter (Ed.), *Minnesota symposium on child psychology* (Vol. 16, pp. 41–83). Hillsdale, NJ: Erlbaum.

Sroufe, L. A., Fox, N. E., & Pancake, V. R. (1983). Attachment and dependency in developmental perspective. *Child Development, 54*, 1615–1627.

Stamler, C., & Palmer, J. O. (1971). Dependency and repetitive visits to the nurse's office in elementary school children. *Nursing Research, 20*, 254–255.

Stangler, R. S., & Printz, A. M. (1980). DSM-III: Psychiatric diagnosis in a university population. *American Journal of Psychiatry, 137*, 937–940.

Stankovic, S. R., Libb, J. W., Freeman, A. M., & Roseman, J. M. (1992). Post-treatment stability of the MCMI—II personality scales in depressed outpatients. *Journal of Personality Disorders, 6*, 82–89.

Steele, R. E. (1978). Relationship of race, sex, social class and social mobility to depression in normal adults. *Journal of Social Psychology, 104*, 37–47.

Stein, N., & Sanfilipo, M. (1985). Depression and the wish to be held. *Journal of Clinical Psychology, 41*, 3–9.

Stendler, C. B. (1954). Possible causes of overdependency in young children. *Child Development, 25*, 125–146.

Stern, R. (1987). *Theories of the unconscious and theories of the self*. Hillsdale, NJ: Erlbaum.

Stewart, S. H., Knize, K., & Pihl, R. O. (1992). Anxiety sensitivity and dependency in clinical and non-clinical panickers and controls. *Journal of Anxiety Disorders, 6*, 119–131.

Stith, M., & Connor, R. (1962). Dependency and helpfulness in young children. *Child Development, 33*, 15–20.

Stores, G., & Piran, N. (1978). Dependency of different types in schoolchildren with epilepsy. *Psychological Medicine, 8*, 441–445.

Strack, S., Lorr, M., & Campbell, L. (1990). An evaluation of Millon's circular model of personality disorders. *Journal of Personality Disorders*, 4, 353–361.

Strack, S., Lorr, M., Campbell, L., & Lamnin, A. (1992). Personality disorder and clinical syndrome factors of MCMI–II scales. *Journal of Personality Disorders*, 6, 40–52.

Strauss, J., & Ryan, R. M. (1987). Autonomy disturbances in subtypes of anorexia nervosa. *Journal of Abnormal Psychology*, 96, 254–258.

Streitfeld, H. S. (1954). Specificity of peptic ulcer to intense oral conflicts. *Psychosomatic Medicine*, 16, 315–326.

Strong, S. R., Welsh, J. A., Corcoran, J. L., & Hoyt, W. T. (1992). Social psychology and counseling psychology: The history, products and promise of an interface. *Journal of Counseling Psychology*, 39, 139–157.

Sullivan, H. S. (1947). *Conceptions of modern psychiatry*. Washington, DC: William Alanson White Institute.

Svanum, S., & Ehrmann, L. C. (1992). Alcoholic subtypes and the MacAndrew Alcoholism Scale. *Journal of Personality Assessment*, 58, 411–422.

Symonds, A. (1971). Phobias after marriage: Women's declaration of dependence. *American Journal of Psychoanalysis*, 31, 144–152.

Symour, N. K. (1977). The dependency cycle. *Transactional Analysis Journal*, 7, 37–43.

Tabachnick, N. (1961). Interpersonal relations in suicide attempts. *Archives of General Psychiatry*, 4, 16–21.

Taccoen, L., & Ansoms, S. (1980). Perceptual dependency, personality structure and organicity in the case of chronic alcoholics. *Acta Psychiatrica Belgica*, 80, 202–219.

Takahashi, K. (1970). Dependency behavior in female adolescents. *Japanese Journal of Educational Psychology*, 18, 65–75.

Talbot, N., Duberstein, P. R., & Scott, P. (1991). Subliminal psychodynamic activation, food consumption and self-confidence. *Journal of Clinical Psychology*, 47, 813–823.

Taylor, R. D., Messick, D. M., Lehman, G. A., & Hirsch, J. K. (1982). Sex, dependency and helping revisited. *Journal of Social Psychology*, 118, 59–65.

Temoshok, L. (1987). Personality, coping style, emotion and cancer. *Cancer Surveys*, 6, 545–567.

Tesser, A., & Blusiewicz, C. O. (1987). Dependency conflict and underachievement. *Journal of Social and Clinical Psychology*, 5, 378–390.

Test, M. A., & Bryan, J. H. (1969). The effects of dependency, models and reciprocity upon subsequent helping behavior. *Journal of Social Psychology*, 28, 205–212.

Thibaut, J. W., & Kelley, H. H. (1959). *The social psychology of groups*. New York: Wiley.

Thomas, A., & Chess, S. (1977). *Temperament and development*. New York: Brunner/Mazel.

Thomas, C. B., & Duszynski, K. R. (1974). Closeness to parents and the family constellation in a prospective study of five disease states. *Johns Hopkins Medical Journal*, 134, 251–270.

Thurston, J. R., & Mussen, P. H. (1951). Infant feeding gratification and adult personality. *Journal of Personality*, *19*, 449–458.

Timmons, E., & Noblin, C. (1963). The differential performance of orals and anals in a verbal conditioning paradigm. *Journal of Consulting Psychology*, *27*, 383–386.

Tisdale, M. J., Pendleton, L., & Marler, M. (1990). MCMI characteristics of DSM-III-R bulimics. *Journal of Personality Assessment*, *55*, 477–483.

Tognazzo, D. P. (1970). Oral Rorschach content in a group of alcoholics. *Psichiatrica Generale e Dell-ete Evolutiva*, *8*, 323–325.

Torgerson, S. (1979). The nature and origin of common phobic fears. *American Journal of Psychiatry*, *134*, 343–351.

Torgerson, S., & Alnaes, R. (1990). The relationship between the MCMI personality scales and DSM-III Axis II. *Journal of Personality Assessment*, *55*, 698–707.

Tribich, D., & Messer, S. (1974). Psychoanalytic character type and status of authority as determiners of suggestibility. *Journal of Consulting and Clinical Psychology*, *42*, 842–848.

Tripathi, N. K. M. (1982). Approval motive and dependence proneness. *Perspectives in Psychological Research*, *5*, 23–28.

Trull, T. J., Widiger, T. A., & Frances, A. (1987). Covariation of criteria sets for avoidant, schizoid and dependent personality disorders. *American Journal of Psychiatry*, *144*, 767–771.

Turkat, I. D., & Carlson, C. R. (1984). Data-based vs. symptomatic formulation of treatment: The case of a dependent personality. *Journal of Behavior Therapy and Experimental Psychiatry*, *15*, 153–160.

Turner, P. J. (1991). Relations between attachment, gender and behavior with peers in preschool. *Child Development*, *62*, 1475–1488.

Vaillant, G. E. (1974). Natural history of male psychological health, II: Some antecedents of healthy adult adjustment. *Archives of General Psychiatry*, *31*, 15–22.

Vaillant, G. E. (1978). Natural history of male psychological health, IV: What kinds of men do not get psychosomatic illness? *Psychosomatic Medicine*, *40*, 420–431.

Vaillant, G. E. (1980). Natural history of male psychological health, VIII: Antecendents of alcoholism and orality. *American Journal of Psychiatry*, *137*, 181–186.

Vaillant, G. E. (1983). *The natural history of alcoholism*. Cambridge, MA: Harvard University Press.

Vandenberg, P., & Helstone, F. (1975). Oral, obsessive and hysterical personality patterns: A Dutch replication. *Journal of Psychiatric Research*, *12*, 319–327.

Vats, A. (1986). Birth order, sex and dependence proneness in Indian students. *Psychological Reports*, *58*, 284–286.

Veldman, D. J., & Brown, O. H. (1969). Personality and performance characteristics associated with cigarette smoking among college freshmen. *Journal of Consulting and Clinical Psychology*, *33*, 109–119.

Vernier, C. M., Barrell, R. P., Cummings, J. W., Dickerson, J. H., & Cooper, H. E. (1961). Psychosocial study of the patient with pulmonary tuberculosis. *Psychological Monographs*, *75* (1, Whole No. 510).

Viederman, M. (1974). Adaptive and maladaptive regression in hemodialysis. *Psychiatry*, *37*, 68–77.

Von Holt, H. W., Sengstake, C. B., Sanada, B. C., & Draper, W. A. (1960). Orality, image fusion and concept formation. *Journal of Projective Techniques*, *24*, 194–198.

Wagner, E. E. (1983). *The Hand Test: Manual for administration, scoring and interpretation*. Los Angeles: Western Psychological Services.

Wallot, H., & Lambert, J. (1984). Characteristics of physician addicts. *American Journal of Drug and Alcohol Abuse*, *10*, 53–62.

Walters, R. H., & Parke, R. D. (1964). Social motivation, dependency and susceptibility to social influence. In L. Berkowitz (Ed.), *Advances in experimental social psychology* (Vol. 1, pp. 231–276). New York: Academic Press.

Waters, E., & Deane, K. E. (1985). Defining and assessing individual differences in attachment relationships. *Monographs of the Society for Research in Child Development*, *50*, 41–65.

Watson, G. (1934). A comparison of the effects of lax versus strict home training. *Journal of Social Psychology*, *5*, 102–105.

Watson, G. (1957). Some personality differences in children related to strict or permissive parental discipline. *Journal of Psychology*, *44*, 227–249.

Watson, P. J., Biderman, M. D., & Boyd, C. (1989). Androgeny as synthetic narcissism: Sex role measures and Kohut's psychology of the self. *Sex Roles*, *21*, 175–207.

Wegscheider-Cruse, S. (1985). *Choicemaking*. Pompano Beach, FL: Health Communications.

Wehler, R. (1979). Attitudes toward mental illness and dependency among hospitalized psychiatric patients. *Psychological Reports*, *44*, 283–286.

Weiner, H., Thaler, M., Reiser, M. E., & Mirsky, I. A. (1957). Etiology of duodenal ulcer, I: Relation of specific psychological characteristics to rate of gastric secretion. *Psychosomatic Medicine*, *19*, 1–10.

Weiss, L. R. (1969). Effects of subject, experimenter and task variables on compliance with the experimenter's expectation. *Journal of Projective Techniques and Personality Assessment*, *33*, 247–256.

Weiss, L. R., & Masling, J. (1970). Further validation of a Rorschach measure of oral imagery: A study of six clinical groups. *Journal of Abnormal Psychology*, *76*, 83–87.

Weiss, P., & Emmerich, W. (1962). Dependency fantasy and group conformity in ulcer patients. *Journal of Consulting Psychology*, *26*, 61–64.

Weiss, R. D., Mirin, S. M., Michael, J. L., & Sollogub, A. C. (1986). Psychopathology in chronic cocaine abusers. *American Journal of Drug and Alcohol Abuse*, *12*, 17–29.

Weissman, A. N., & Beck, A. T. (1978). *Development and validation of the Dysfunctional Attitudes Scale*. Paper presented at the American Educational Research Association Meeting, Toronto, Canada.

Welkowitz, J., Lish, J. D., & Bond, R. N. (1985). The Depressive Experiences Questionnaire: Revision and validation. *Journal of Personality Assessment*, *49*, 89–94.

West, M., Livesley, W. J., Reiffer, L., & Sheldon, A. (1986). The place of attachment in the life events model of stress and illness. *Canadian Journal of Psychiatry, 31*, 202–207.

Westen, D. (1991). Social cognition and object relations. *Psychological Bulletin, 109*, 429–455.

Whiffen, V. E., & Sasseville, T. M. (1991). Dependency, self-criticism and recollections of parenting: Sex differences and the role of depressive affect. *Journal of Social and Clinical Psychology, 10*, 121–133.

White, H. (1986). Damsels in distress: Dependency themes in fiction for children and adolescents. *Adolescence, 21*, 251–256.

Whiting, J. W. M. (1944). The frustration complex in Kwoma society. *Man, 44*, 140–144.

Whiting, J. W. M., & Child, I. (1953). *Child training and personality*. New Haven, CT: Yale University Press.

Wickstrom, D. L., & Fleck, J. R. (1983). Missionary children: Correlates of self-esteem and dependency. *Journal of Psychology and Theology, 11*, 226–235.

Widiger, T. A., Freiman, K., & Bailey, B. (1990). Convergent and discriminant validity of personality disorder prototypic acts. *Psychological Assessment, 2*, 107–113.

Widiger, T. A., & Sanderson, C. (1987). The convergent and discriminant validity of the MCMI as a measure of DSM-III personality disorders. *Journal of Personality Assessment, 51*, 228–242.

Widiger, T. A., & Spitzer, R. L. (1991). Sex bias in the diagnosis of personality disorders: Conceptual and methodological issues. *Clinical Psychology Review, 11*, 1–22.

Widiger, T. A., Williams, J. B. W., Spitzer, R. L., & Frances, A. (1985). The MCMI as a measure of DSM-III. *Journal of Personality Assessment, 49*, 366–378.

Wiener, G. (1956). Neurotic depressives and alcoholics: Oral Rorschach percepts. *Journal of Projective Techniques, 20*, 534–455.

Wiggins, J. S., & Winder, C. L. (1961). The Peer Nomination Inventory. *Psychological Reports, 9*, 643–677.

Wilke, H., & Lanzetta, J. T. (1982). The obligation to help: Factors affecting response to help received. *European Journal of Social Psychology, 12*, 315–319.

Wilkin, D. (1987). Conceptual problems in dependency research. *Social Science and Medicine, 24*, 867–873.

Williams, J. S. (1975). Aspects of dependence–independence conflict in children with asthma. *Journal of Child Psychology and Psychiatry, 16*, 199–218.

Wilson, K. E., & Shantz, C. U. (1977). Perceptual role-taking ability and dependency behavior in preschool children. *Merrill-Palmer Quarterly, 23*, 207–211.

Winder, C. L., Ahmad, F. Z., Bandura, A., & Rau, L. (1962). Dependency of patients, psychotherapists' responses, and aspects of psychotherapy. *Journal of Consulting Psychology, 26*, 129–134.

Winder, C. L., & Rau, L. (1962). Parental attitudes associated with social deviance in preadolescent boys. *Journal of Abnormal and Social Psychology, 64*, 418–424.

Wittenborn, J. R. (1956). A study of adoptive children: Relationship between some aspects of development and some aspects of environment for adoptive children. *Psychological Monographs, 70* (Whole No. 410).

Wittenborn, J. R., & Maurer, H. S. (1977). Persistent personalities among depressed women. *Archives of General Psychiatry, 34,* 968–971.

Wold, P. N. (1983). Anorexic syndromes and affective disorder. *Psychiatric Journal of the University of Ottawa, 8,* 116–119.

Wolfson, S. L. (1981). Sex, dependency and volunteering. *British Journal of Social Psychology, 20,* 293–294.

Wolowitz, H. M. (1967). Oral involvement in peptic ulcer. *Journal of Consulting Psychology, 31,* 418–419.

Wolowitz, H. M., & Barker, M. J. (1968). Alcoholism and oral passivity. *Quarterly Journal of Studies on Alcohol, 29,* 592–597.

Wolowitz, H. M., & Wagonfeld, S. (1968). Oral derivatives in the food preferences of peptic ulcer patients. *Journal of Nervous and Mental Disease, 146,* 18–23.

Wonderlich, S. A., Swift, W. J., Slotnick, H. B., & Goodman, S. (1990). DSM-III-R personality disorders in eating disorder subtypes. *International Journal of Eating Disorders, 9,* 607–616.

Woolams, S. J., & Huige, K. A. (1977). Normal dependency and symbiosis. *Transactional Analysis Journal, 7,* 217–220.

Yager, J., Landsverk, J., Edelstein, C. K., & Hyler, S. E. (1989). Screening for Axis II personality disorders in women with bulimic eating disorders. *Psychosomatics, 30,* 255–262.

Yasunaga, S. (1985). The effects of dependency and strategy patterns on modeling. *Japanese Journal of Psychology, 55,* 374–377.

Yeger, T., & Miezitis, S. (1985). Pupil sex as it relates to the pupil–teacher dependency relationship. *International Journal of Women's Studies, 8,* 457–464.

Young, J. Y., & Smith, A. B. (1977). Dependency behavior as related to separation in a day-care setting. *New Zealand Journal of Educational Studies, 12,* 57–63.

Zeldow, P. B., & Greenberg, R. P. (1979). Attitudes toward women and orientation to seeking professional help. *Journal of Clinical Psychology, 35,* 473–476.

Zeldow, P. B., & Greenberg, R. P. (1980). Who goes where: Sex differences in psychological and medical help seeking. *Journal of the American Psychiatric Association, 44,* 433–435.

Zimmerman, M., & Coryell, W. (1989). DSM-III personality disorder diagnoses in a nonpatient sample. *Archives of General Psychiatry, 46,* 682–689.

Zirkel, S. (1992). Developing independence in a life transition: Investing the self in the concerns of the day. *Journal of Personality and Social Psychology, 62,* 506–521.

Zuckerman, M. (1958). The validity of the Edwards Personal Preference Schedule in the measurement of dependency–rebelliousness. *Journal of Clinical Psychology, 14,* 379–382.

Zuckerman, M., & Grosz, H. J. (1958). Suggestibility and dependency. *Journal of Consulting Psychology, 22,* 328.

Zuckerman, M., Levitt, E. E., & Lubin, B. (1961). Concurrent and construct validity of direct and indirect measures of dependency. *Journal of Consulting Psychology, 25,* 316–323.

Zung, W. W. K. (1965). A self-rating depression scale. *Archives of General Psychiatry, 12,* 63–70.

Zuroff, D. C., & DeLorimier, S. (1989). Ideal and actual romantic partners of women varying in dependency and self-criticism. *Journal of Personality*, *57*, 825–846.

Zuroff, D. C., Igreja, I., & Mongrain, M. (1990). Dysfunctional attitudes, dependency and self-criticism as predictors of depressive mood states: A 12–month longitudinal study. *Cognitive Therapy and Research*, *14*, 315–326.

Zuroff, D. C., & Mongrain, M. (1987). Dependency and self-criticism: Vulnerability factors for depressive affective states. *Journal of Abnormal Psychology*, *96*, 14–22.

Zuroff, D. C., Moskowitz, D. S., Wielgus, M. S., Powers, T. A., & Franko, D. L. (1983). Construct validation of the dependency and self-criticism scales of the Depressive Experiences Questionnaire. *Journal of Research in Personality*, *17*, 226–241.

# Author Index

# Subject Index

234